Outwitting Insomnia

Overcoming Sleeplessness and Getting the Rest You Need with Classic and Cutting-Edge Remedies That Really Work

Ellen Mohr Catalano

Series Concept Created by Bill Adler, Jr.

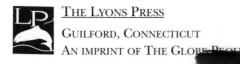

THE LYONS PRESS
GUILFORD, CONNECTICUT
AN IMPRINT OF THE GLOBE PEQUOT PRESS

The Lyons Press is an imprint of The Globe Pequot Press.

10 9 8 7 6 5 4 3 2 1

Printed in the United States of America

ISBN 1-59228-123-0

Library of Congress Cataloging-in-Publication Data is available on file.

Contents

Acknowledgments

I wish to thank the following people for their time and updated information: Dr. Gene Block, Vice President and Provost of the University of Virginia; Dr. Mark E. Williams, Director of Geriatric Services at the University of Virginia; Catherine Zuver, RN, of the Women's Midlife Health Center at the University of Virginia; Dr. Charles Morin of the Université Laval, Quebec, Canada; Dr. Sandy Grammling of the Psychology Department at Virginia Commonwealth University, Richmond, Virginia; Dr. James K. Walsh of the Sleep Medicine and Research Center in Chesterfield, Missouri, for his authorship of the medications chapter in the original book; Dr. Nancy Union of Charlottesville, Virginia, for her information on acupuncture; and Paul Olko, also of Charlottesville, for his knowledge of Chinese Medicine. A huge, heartfelt thanks goes to the "genies" in my life, Jean Martin Johnson and Jeannie Siler, who created magic with their expert editing. And finally, grateful thanks to my friends and family, especially to my husband, Glenn, and our daughter, Rubina, for patiently supporting me and enduring the predictable ups and downs of reproducing a book.

Introduction

This book first appeared almost thirteen years ago. I think of who I was thirteen years ago and am amazed to think of how innocently I slept and took that sleep for granted. A complete night of sound, restful Z's were almost always available back then. And if I couldn't sleep, it was usually due to random occurrences of pre-exam jitters or holiday excitement.

Since then the world has changed at a startling rate: burgeoning access to the internet, increased threats of terrorism, seemingly random viruses that spread worldwide, and more. While you might think sleep is sleep, no matter what era we live in, you are only partially right. Our understanding of the basic mechanism of sleep remains the same, with the body needing about seven to eight hours of quality rest per night. Factors affecting sleep also remain similar, such as diet, exercise, and sleep hygiene. Anxiety, as usual, remains a prevalent influence on insomnia. So, the reasons people had trouble sleeping then were in many ways exactly the same as now, with some critical differences. For example, the bar on our health status is significantly raised when you factor in such pressures as terrorism, our economy, an aging population, and near-instant access to worldwide information. Certainly not least in these factors is the horrific fact that our country has been attacked on its own soil for the first time in sixty years. The resultant heightened security has essentially infiltrated everyone's homes and families, and fear for our safety is enough to cause anyone restless, if not totally sleepless, nights.

The National Sleep Federation (NSF), an independent nonprofit organization, has been annually collecting statistics on how people sleep. The results of its 2002 *Sleep in America* poll show what may be a trend toward less sleep. Fewer adults appear to be getting eight or more hours of sleep each night compared to the previous year (38 percent versus 30 percent). Overall, 24 percent reported that they got less than the minimum amount of sleep they believed they needed to not feel sleepy the next day. NSF's 2003 poll showed that almost half of all adults surveyed (48 percent of adults fifty-five to eighty-four years old) report having one or more symptoms of insomnia at least a few nights per week.

No matter what the age, Americans as a group are staying up later and getting up earlier, reports the *Wall Street Journal* (April 1, 2003). Over the last decade or so, people have cut their sleep by an hour on average, in part because of the availability of technology such as e-mail and in part because of the age-old problem of stress. Healthology, Inc., a producer and distributor of physician-generated health and medical information on the internet reports, "Because of lack of sleep, approximately $90 billion per year is spent on lost productivity, absenteeism at work, car accidents and sleep and stimulant medication."

Since the boomers are aging rapidly, our national attention deservedly turns to all the concomitant problems aging can cause. According to an article from the Centers for Disease Control on public health and aging the number of people sixty-five and over is expected to increase from approximately thirty-five million in 2000 to an estimated seventy-one million in 2030. In fact, worldwide, the average life span is expected to extend another ten years by 2050. Throw into this mix the potentially negative effects of ceasing hormone replacement therapy (HRT). What was once thought to be a reliable sleep aid for all the female boomers is now being seriously questioned. Those who chose to rely on HRT to get them through the night are now left wondering how much sleep they can do without.

As a result of all these external and internal pressures, it became time to update this book and take a fresh look at sleep. We can no longer say that sleep is something many of us take for granted. We can't sleep the sleep of children anymore, although some research is showing that even children and teenagers are sleeping less well these days, suffering from piles of homework and other school-related anxieties.

The problem of getting enough quality sleep exists in young to old and in-between. The only "beings" I can think of that appear to be immune to insomnia are cats and dogs. One reason I like having my furry pals around me is that they always appear to be blissfully comfortable wherever they are, whether napping or settled in for the night. Just watching them curled up can be a tonic for my frazzled self.

But back to humans. There is encouraging news out there for insomnia sufferers since this book was first written. Effective non-addictive medications for sleep have emerged to take the place of the Valium class of addictive drugs. Exercise, always a recommended tonic for the hectic, remains strongly encouraged. More is known about the medical causes underlying sleep disorders such as sleep apnea. The accessibility of the internet provides an almost overwhelming array of choices from herbals, gadgets, and gizmos to help you sleep better, to the nearest sleep center. That said, I've taken the time to weed through the internet pop-up ads and other Web sites to provide you with a list of reliable addresses where you can gather new ideas and information. At the end of the book is an appendix containing pertinent internet addresses along with other references. And speaking of the Web, if anything, the internet can offer you endless late-night company via chat rooms. It's nice to know that you never have to face a cold dark house in the middle of the night all alone. Grab a steamy hot mug of something and cozy up to the screen in your warm bathrobe— and visit your internet pals.

Some chapters are new additions to the original edition, such as the chapter on menopause and sleep. I sincerely thank contributor and reviewer Mary Evans, MD, formally a health writer for the Mayo Clinic, for providing us with an in-depth look at the complex issues of menopause, insomnia, and HRT. As women seek to rely less on HRT and explore alternative medicine, I've added a chapter on Complementary and Alternative Medicine (CAM). Many thanks to Shalom Vegodsky, herbalist and naturopath, for her review and current information. Also included in this chapter is a description of acupuncture and its healing effects on the body. Dr. Jeff Jenkins of the University of Virginia's Physical Medicine and Rehabilitation contributes his expertise to describe acupuncture's basic concepts, and why it would have potentially beneficial effects on insomnia.

Contributor and reviewer Mary Preston, MD, an expert on aging at the University of Virginia, gives us an updated review of common medications prescribed for insomnia and the effects of aging on sleep. She also provides us with a fresh look at the increasing evidence of sleep apnea in the elderly, along with other parasomnias such as restless leg syndrome and REM Behavior Syndrome (RBD). Finally, many thanks to psychologist Phyllis Koch-Sheras, author and expert on dreaming, for her updated information and review of dreams and sleep.

Those are the highlights of new and/or updated portions of the book; other time-honored best sleep practices remain, such as healthy sleep hygiene, meditation, and relaxation techniques— all equally important in their basic contribution to what helps us sleep. We also continue to thank the original authors of the sleep and chronic pain chapter, Charles Morin, Ph.D., and Sandy Grammling, Ph.D. Sleep is obviously influenced by pain; their comprehensive approach offers common sense advice for dealing with a major disruptor of sleep.

Sleep is something you once took for granted, like breathing. In childhood it was as natural as being hungry. Why does sleep change as you age? What can you do in adulthood to find restful sleep, to reprogram yourself to shed daytime worries so you can re-create the sleep experienced as a child?

Part of the answer lies in awareness and in an understanding of your unique self. As with undertaking any behavioral change, the first step is for you to set aside previously held beliefs and familiar rituals about sleep. Adopt an open mind-set; question your assumptions. Make it a habit to do a self-check to see if you are closing your mind to the possibilities. If you follow the suggestions in the chapters ahead, you can have faith that you will find ways to improve your sleep significantly and permanently.

About Insomnia

Sophie dreads crawling into bed each night. She's tried counting sheep and imagining ocean waves, only to find that her mind wanders back to the anxieties of the day. She struggles for a good hour in bed, but sleep eludes her. She looks at the clock repeatedly, a brightly lit digital thing that details precisely how much time has passed. This, of course, only makes her more anxious. She says things to herself like, "If I don't go to sleep *now* I will *never* be able to make it through tomorrow." Sophie suffers from a very common type of insomnia, trouble falling asleep, sometimes known as *sleep onset insomnia*.

Leah, on the other hand, falls asleep quickly. But after a couple of hours she becomes restless and wakes up. If she falls back asleep, she wakes up again, two or three times throughout the night. On some nights she cannot force herself to go back to sleep at all, and so spends the next day haggard and cranky. Leah suffers from *sleep maintenance insomnia,* or staying asleep throughout the night.

David is out the moment his head hits the pillow. His sleeping companion assures him he's snoring *loudly* in seconds. He sleeps soundly until around 3 A.M. or 4 A.M., when he abruptly awakes, mind racing. David suffers from *waking up too early,* a third type of insomnia. What's worse, all his thoughts, no matter how trivial they look in daylight, seem absolutely catastrophic in the wee hours.

Eddie feels that he gets an adequate amount of sleep every night, but still feels a great deal of fatigue the next day. In fact, he wakes up tired with stiff and sore muscles, but visits to the doctor do not reveal any particular disease process such as arthritis. His condition is called *nonrestorative sleep*.

These four types of insomnia are common examples of the wide array of problems that can plague your sleep. In fact, the American Sleep Disorders Association currently recognizes seventy-eight different sleep disorders described in the *International Classification of Sleep Disorders*.

Perhaps a more useful way to think about insomnia is to categorize it as simply "transient" or "persistent." Transient, or acute, insomnia is occasional and usually due to stress, environmental factors, or travel across time zones. You may be going through a particularly difficult time in your life and experience bouts of poor quality sleep. You can probably identify an event or events that triggered your anxious reaction. As the stress subsides, so does the insomnia.

When you experience poor sleep over a longer period, at least two to three months, you may have developed persistent or chronic insomnia. Your sleep problem may have started out as transient insomnia, but due to lifestyle habits or an underlying disease process, it developed into a longer-term problem. You need to take care that your persistent insomnia does not involve a medical condition, such as sleep apnea. Refer to chapter 12 for more information about physical disorders and sleep.

You may share some or all of the characteristics described above. Most insomniacs do not fit neatly into any of these specific categories, but exhibit a wide variety of tendencies based on age, heredity, personality, and sleep requirements. For example, you may feel that you require less sleep than other people. Some "short sleepers" experience no disruption in functioning after only four hours of sleep, while others who feel they are "long sleepers" may feel exhausted after nine. If you consider yourself a short sleeper, you share the nighttime hours with such famous people as Margaret Thatcher who was once quoted as saying, "Sleep is for wimps." Or, you may agree with Thomas Edison's disregard for sleep when he said it was a "waste of time." His light bulb invention, while obviously a modern miracle, enables us to work long into the night!

How's Your Sleep?

CHECK IF ANY OF THE FOLLOWING APPLY TO YOU

❑ Snore loudly

❑ You or others have observed that you stop breathing or gasp for breath during sleep

❑ Feel sleepy or doze off while watching TV, reading, driving, or engaged in daily activities

❑ Have difficulty sleeping 3 nights a week or more *(e.g., trouble falling asleep, wake frequently during the night, wake too early and cannot get back to sleep or wake unrefreshed)*

❑ Feel unpleasant, tingling, creeping feelings or nervousness in your legs when trying to sleep

❑ Interruptions to your sleep *(e.g., nighttime heartburn, bad dreams, pain, discomfort, noise, sleep difficulties of family members, light or temperature)*

Sleep Problems are a Serious Threat to Your Health, Safety and Well-Being.

If you have checked one or more of the statements provided, you should make an appointment to discuss this with

your doctor. Please see the information provided below in response to your selection to learn why you may have a sleep problem and what it means.

Snore loudly
Snoring occurs when there is a partial blockage of the airway. Snoring has been linked to increased blood pressure and may be a sign of sleep apnea.

You or others have observed that you stop breathing or gasp for breath during sleep
Observed pauses in breathing, often accompanied by snoring, are a symptom of a serious condition called sleep apnea. These breathing pauses reduce blood-oxygen levels, strain the heart and cardiovascular system, and contribute to daytime sleepiness.

Feel sleepy or doze off while watching TV, reading, driving or engaged in daily activities
Sleepiness during the day or at times when you expect to be awake and alert is a sign that you may be suffering from sleep deprivation, a sleep disorder such as sleep apnea or narcolepsy, or another treatable medical condition. Daytime sleepiness puts you at risk for driving drowsy, injury and illness, and can significantly impair your mental abilities, emotions and performance.

Have difficulty sleeping 3 nights a week or more
Experiencing any of these insomnia symptoms a few nights a week is not a normal sleep pattern. Untreated insomnia is a risk factor for the onset of depression and can jeopardize your emotional outlook, social relations and sense of well-being. The toll of sleep loss can also affect

your health, your safety and your performance in all areas of life.

Feel unpleasant, tingling, creeping feelings or nervousness in your legs when trying to sleep
These feelings in your legs indicate that you may have Restless Legs Syndrome (RLS), a neurological movement disorder characterized by a strong urge to move the legs and difficulty falling and staying asleep.

Interruptions to your sleep
Disruptions compromise both the quantity and quality of sleep and keep you from experiencing continuous, restorative sleep so necessary for performance, safety, and health. They can be caused by an acute or chronic medical condition, a bright, noisy, or uncomfortable environment, or awakenings caused by other people. Determining the causes of any sleep disruptions will help you and your doctor determine the best treatment.

(Reprinted with permission from the National Sleep Foundation.)

Most people, however, require an average of eight hours of quality sleep per night. By quality, we mean passing through the normal stages of sleep. Sleep progresses from lighter to deeper stages in a cyclic pattern, repeated throughout the night. The NSF refers to these cycles as a "dynamic process with a complex architecture all its own." This architecture is displayed in the form of brain waves emitted at each of the sleep stages. Scientists can measure these waves in a sleep lab by means of a machine called an electroencephalograph (EEG). The waves depict a person's progression through a typical night of sleep. For example, you emit beta waves when awake doing normal activity. Alpha waves are associated with calm wakefulness, such as when you sit down, take a break, or right as you close your eyes to sleep. As soon as you actually fall asleep, you enter stage 1 of sleep, where theta waves are measured. After about 5 minutes of stage 1, stage 2 begins, which emit waves called sleep spindles and K complexes. Stage 2 lasts for only 5–10 more minutes, at which point you enter stages 3 and 4 of sleep known as the deepest stages, where delta waves are emitted. Following Delta, or Slow Wave Sleep (SWS), are the periods of sleep associated with Rapid Eye Movement (REM). You cycle through these stages throughout the night, and the fine points and distinctions of each stage are still being debated by scientists. But one thing is certain: You need all of these stages for healthy and restorative sleep, and the amount of time you spend in each stage is not as important as that your sleep be continuous and un-fragmented.

Getting a sufficient amount of sleep each night requires that you pass through all of these cycles, with minimal interruptions if possible. Interruptions are hard to avoid, however, with our twenty-four-hour access to artificial light, shopping, and the internet, not to mention work and family demands and the effects of aging on our quality of sleep. You may also experience disturbed sleep if you abuse substances, work night shifts, and take long naps during the day. More about sleep hygiene, or good sleep practices, in the next chapter. The NSF urges us to keep in mind that in the past century, we have reduced our average time asleep by 20 percent, and, in the past twenty-five years, added a month to our average annual work/commute time. Sleep Guru Dr. William Dement calls us a "sleep-sick society." And the cost is high. Healthology, a Web site offering physician-generated health and medical information on the internet reports that because of lack of sleep, approximately $90 billion per year is spent on lost productivity, absenteeism at work, car accidents, and sleep and stimulant medication.

Human need for sleep changes with age. Newborn babies sleep about two thirds of the time, decreasing to about 50 percent, or twelve hours per night, at six months of age. Children continue to sleep about ten to twelve hours per night, leveling off at seven and one-half hours per night with teenagers and adults. By age fifty-five, the hours of sleep increase to eight or more again, but the sleep quality is different. Aged sleep tends to be lighter and more restless, with a typical number of awakenings at five per night. This can be a natural function of age, but it frightens some people into thinking they are suffering from insomnia. Insomnia is not necessarily an outcome of aging, but could be the result of chronic illness or depression. More about aging and sleep in chapter 10.

The following widely used, multifaceted guidelines can help you identify insomnia. If nearly all the conditions match your experience, you suffer persistent insomnia. Any one symptom, however, can indicate sleep problems significant enough to disrupt functioning and warrant your attention.

1. Taking more than thirty minutes to fall asleep
2. Being awake more than a total of thirty minutes during the night, or
3. Sleeping less than a total of six and one-half hours
4. Experiencing daytime fatigue with decreased performance ability and increased moodiness
5. Symptoms occurring three or more nights per week for one month or more

Insomnia can be caused, and prolonged by, any of the following:

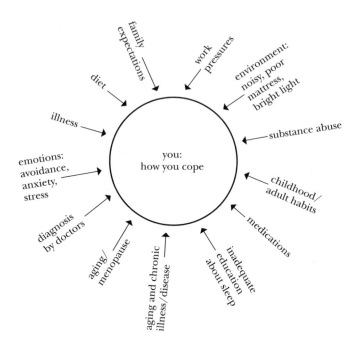

In the center of the diagram is "how you cope." Coping encompasses physical as well as emotional adjustment. You probably already know that being physically tense hinders your ability to relax enough to go to sleep. Insomniacs are known to be people with a history of general physical arousal, meaning that they tense up easily and stay tensed for prolonged periods. This may mean higher muscle tension and blood pressure, faster heart rate, and poorer peripheral circulation. To make matters worse, all of these tendencies are exacerbated when you are under stress, creating a vicious cycle of anxiety—sleeplessness—more anxiety. If you know that you are the type of person who easily tenses up—your muscles are sore from tension and fatigue or you are prone to headaches—you will likely benefit from the relaxation exercises presented in chapter 3. Most insomniacs respond best, however, to a combination of relaxation exercises and cognitive control of their obsessive thinking.

Nine Psycho-physiological Factors Involved in Insomnia

It is impossible to make a complete list of all the factors shared by insomniacs. With 30 percent to 40 percent of the adult population reporting some degree of insomnia, the group is enormously diverse, and the problem is unique for each individual. Nevertheless, some general tendencies link insomniacs. The fact that these characteristics involve both the mind as well as the body is strong testimony to the importance of managing your emotional, as well as physical, self.

Insomniacs as a group tend to have certain emotional characteristics that keep them from sleep. One primary characteristic is "fear of letting go." Insomniacs have trouble letting go not only of physical tension but also of thoughts. Do you find that you have difficulty accepting that a problem is not solvable? Can you say to yourself, "Let it go," and believe it? Your inability to let thoughts and feelings go leads to "obsessive thinking." You may catch yourself lying in bed at night obsessing about everything from potential personal failures to solving the world's problems. You may often feel a great deal of anger at yourself and others, and insecurity, and then blame yourself for not being perfect. These perfectionistic tendencies create destructive, circular patterns: you get angry, place blame, can't get to sleep, and then get angry with yourself for being so weak that you can't get to sleep. In summary, the nine typical characteristics are:

1. high physical arousal levels
2. fear of letting go
3. obsessional thinking
4. fear of failure

5. anger
6. catastrophic thinking
7. perfectionistic tendencies
8. participation in vicious cycle patterns
9. letting anxious thoughts control you

If any or all of these nine thought and behavior patterns sound familiar, take heart. There are ways to counteract their negative effects, which interfere with your sleep. Chapters 6 and 7 describe relaxation techniques you can use to calm your tense body. Chapter 8 goes into greater detail about specific techniques to manage your obsessive thinking and counteract the negative energy that only makes it harder for you to cope.

Summary

It's lonely being an insomniac. No one else—no doctor, parent, friend, or even spouse—can give you a magic cure to help you sleep. A cure, that is, that is healthy, practical, inexpensive, and nonaddictive. What's worse, you face most of those feelings of isolation and frustration in the middle of the night, when others are snoozing peacefully. That's when you're likely to feel most resentful of others' ability to sleep. That's also when you probably obsess about all the things you think you're doing wrong in your life. You might even be tempted to lash out angrily at others and—directly or indirectly—blame them for your insomnia. You may wish or even insist that your significant other wakes to share your misery. Resist this temptation; a friend doesn't need to share sleepless nights to sympathize with you. Chances are she already feels helpless and anxious about your condition.

This book is designed as a self-help guide to treatment. The exercises and ideas presented in these pages can help you identify and gain control over your sleep problems. Nevertheless, you may choose to have yourself evaluated by a certified professional in a sleep lab to ensure that you are not overlooking a serious health problem. A professional evaluation also offers you an individualized, detailed profile of your condition. Chapter 11, "Sleep and Chronic Pain," contains a description and discussion of the sleep lab experience.

Sleep IQ Test

Think you're a sleep genius? In a 1999 nationwide survey, 83 percent of adult Americans failed the NSF Sleep IQ Test. The average person gave fewer than six correct responses. Find out your sleep IQ by taking the test below.

True   False

❑   ❑   1. During sleep, your brain rests.

❑   ❑   2. You cannot learn to function normally with one or two fewer hours of sleep a night than you need.

❑   ❑   3. Boredom makes you feel sleepy, even if you have had enough sleep.

❑   ❑   4. Resting in bed with your eyes closed cannot satisfy your body's need for sleep.

❑   ❑   5. Snoring is not harmful as long as it doesn't disturb others or wake you up.

❑   ❑   6. Everyone dreams every night.

❑   ❑   7. The older you get, the fewer hours of sleep you need.

❏	❏	8. Most people don't know when they are sleepy.
❏	❏	9. Raising the volume of your radio will help you stay awake while driving.
❏	❏	10. Sleep disorders are mainly due to worry or psychological problems.
❏	❏	11. The human body never adjusts to night shift work.
❏	❏	12. Most sleep disorders go away even without treatment.

What's My Sleep IQ?

1. *During sleep, your brain rests.*
   False. While your body rests, your brain doesn't. An active brain during sleep prepares us for alertness and peak functioning the next day.

2. *You cannot learn to function normally with one or two fewer hours of sleep a night than you need.*
   True. Sleep need is biological. While children need more sleep than adults, how much sleep any individual needs is genetically determined. Most adults need eight hours of sleep to function at their best. How to determine what you need? Sleep until you wake on your own . . . without an alarm clock. Feel rested? That's your sleep need. You can teach yourself to sleep less, but not to need less sleep.

3. *Boredom makes you feel sleepy, even if you have had enough sleep.*
   False. When people are active, they usually don't feel sleepy. When they take a break from activity, or feel bored, they may notice that they are sleepy. However,

what causes sleepiness most is sleep loss: not getting the sleep you need. Adults who don't get enough good sleep feel sleepy when they're bored. Boredom, like a warm or dark room, doesn't cause sleepiness, it merely unmasks it.

4. *Resting in bed with your eyes closed cannot satisfy your body's need for sleep.*
True. Sleep is as necessary to health as food and water, and rest is no substitute for sleep. As noted above, sleep is an active process needed for health and alertness. When you don't get the sleep you need, your body builds up a sleep debt. Sooner or later, this debt must be paid . . . with sleep. If you drive when you're sleepy, you place yourself and others at risk because drowsy drivers can fall asleep at the wheel with little or no warning. Sleepiness contributes to driver inattention, which is related to one million crashes each year!

5. *Snoring is not harmful as long as it doesn't disturb others or wake you up.*
False. Snoring may indicate the presence of a life-threatening sleep disorder called sleep apnea. People with sleep apnea snore loudly and arouse repeatedly during the night, gasping for breath. These repeated awakenings lead to severe daytime sleepiness, which raises the risk for accidents and heart problems. Yet 95 percent of those with sleep apnea remain unaware that they have a serious disorder. The good news: With treatment, patients can improve their sleep and alertness, and reduce their risk for accidents and health problems. Physicians and sleep specialists should be consulted.

6. *Everyone dreams every night.*
   True. Though many people fail to remember their dreams, dreaming does occur for every person, every night. Dreams are most vivid during **REM** or rapid eye movement sleep.

7. *The older you get, the fewer hours of sleep you need.*
   False. Sleep need remains unchanged throughout adulthood. Older people may wake more frequently through the night and may sleep less, but their sleep need is no less than during young adulthood. When older people sleep less at night, they tend to sleep more during the day. Sleep difficulties are not a normal part of aging, although they are all too common. If poor sleep habits, pain, or health conditions make sleeping difficult, a physician can help.

8. *Most people don't know when they are sleepy.*
   True. Most people don't know when they're sleepy. Researchers have asked thousands of people over the years if they're sleepy, only to be told no . . . just before the individuals fell asleep! What does this mean? Many people don't know if they are sleepy, when they are sleepy, or why they are sleepy. When driving, don't think you can tough it out if you're sleepy but only a few miles from your destination. If you're sleepy enough, you can fall asleep . . . anywhere.

9. *Raising the volume of your radio will help you stay awake while driving.*
   False. If you're having trouble staying awake while driving, the only short-term solution is to pull over at a safe place and take a short nap or have a caffeinated

drink. Doing both—for example, drinking coffee, then napping before the caffeine kicks in—may be even better. However, the only long-term solution is prevention . . . starting out well rested after a good night's sleep. Research shows that loud radios, chewing gum, and open windows fail to keep sleepy drivers alert.

10. *Sleep disorders are mainly due to worry or psychological problems.*
    False. Stress is the number one reason people report insomnia. However, stress accounts for only a fraction of the people who suffer either chronic insomnia or difficulty staying alert during the day. Sleep disorders have a variety of causes. Sleep apnea, for example, is caused by an obstruction of the airway during sleep. Narcolepsy, which is characterized by severe daytime sleepiness and sudden sleep attacks, appears to be genetic. No one knows yet what causes restless legs syndrome, in which creepy, crawly feelings arise in the legs and are relieved, momentarily, by motion.

11. *The human body never adjusts to night shift work.*
    True. All living things (people, animals, even plants) have a circadian or about 24-hour rhythm. This affects when we feel sleepy and alert. Light and dark cycles set these circadian rhythms. When you travel across time zones, your circadian rhythm adjusts when the light and dark cycle changes. For shift workers, the light and dark cycle doesn't change. Therefore, a shift worker's circadian rhythm never adjusts. Whether you work the night shift or not, you are most likely to feel

sleepy between midnight and six A.M. And no matter how many years one works a night shift, sleeping during the day remains difficult. Shift workers should avoid caffeine during the last half of their workdays, block out noise and light at bedtime, and stay away from alcohol and alerting activities before going to sleep.

12. *Most sleep disorders go away even without treatment.*
False. Unfortunately, many people who suffer from sleep disorders don't realize that they have a disorder or that it can be treated. But sleep disorders don't disappear without treatment. Treatment may be behavioral (for example, going to sleep and waking at the same time every day, scheduling naps or losing weight), pharmacological (involving medication), surgical, or a combination. Untreated sleep disorders may have serious negative effects, worsening quality of life, school and work performance, and relationships. Worse, untreated sleep disorders may lead to accidents and death.

(Reprinted with permission from the National Sleep Foundation.)

Sleep Hygiene

2

In your quest to unravel your sleep problem, you may unknowingly overlook the obvious. Sometimes sleep problems are not related to complex physical or mental disorders, but are simply the
result of poor habits. However, before you decide that your sleep
problem fits into the category of "simple," it's a good idea to consult a sleep expert. As you will see in the chapter on sleep disorders, certain sleep problems such as sleep apnea are serious
enough to require immediate medical attention. If you suspect
you have a physical disorder, you'll want to consult a sleep expert
or reputable health-care practitioner. If you're not sure where
to go, check out the Web site listing for the American Academy
of Sleep Medicine in the appendix for a sleep center near you.
Happily, sleep disorder clinics have proliferated throughout the
United States in the last decade.

In the meantime, consider your sleep hygiene, or sleep habits.
Sometimes the simplest things can get in the way of good sleep.
Throughout this chapter, scrutinize the habits you keep surrounding your up times and down times to see which ones may
need altering. The first part of this chapter will help you consider
your personal habits and pre-bed rituals such as diet, exercise, and
time scheduling. In the second part, you can examine possible

environmental factors that might significantly affect sleep quality, such as noise. A sample sleep diary is included at the end of this chapter; making copies and filling them in regularly can help you isolate significant factors and monitor your progress.

Personal Habits and Pre-Bed Rituals

Diet

Caffeine

One obvious food substance to avoid is caffeine. You probably know someone who brags about drinking coffee all day and then sleeping soundly all night. Chances are that person's sleep is affected more than she realizes. Caffeine is a powerful stimulant; most people will recognize the uncomfortable shakiness and general arousal of even small amounts of caffeine. In large doses, it can cause sweating, heart racing, numbness, breathing difficulties, and paranoid feelings. Caffeine is a drug; you can develop a tolerance, but it will always act as a stimulant. Ingesting anything with caffeine in it even several hours before bedtime can cause difficulty falling asleep and fitful sleep long into the night. Do not drink caffeinated beverages after 4 P.M., or within six hours of your bedtime. If you can cut it out entirely, so much the better. Remember to check the labels on colas, teas, and some other drinks that may contain more caffeine than you realize. Some medications and foods, such as chocolate, contain caffeine. Appendix B lists the caffeine content of many common foods, beverages, and over-the-counter drugs.

Some people get a headache upon abruptly discontinuing caffeine. If you go a day without caffeine and notice a dull persistent headache, you might consider trying "light" coffee at first, or half the caffeine. Simply mix a pound of decaf with a pound of regular.

Nicotine

Like caffeine, nicotine is also a powerful stimulant. Sleep lab studies show that smokers averaging one and one-half packs a day take longer to fall asleep than nonsmokers. Smokers also tend to experience more fitful sleep, which can be worsened by smoker's cough. The health hazards of smoking are well known, and insomnia sufferers should seriously consider giving up their smoking habit for reasons besides improved sleep. If this is simply not an option right now, try not to smoke within two to three hours of your bedtime.

Be aware that abrupt withdrawal of these central nervous system stimulants can have adverse effects. Some people experience headaches, restlessness, and feelings of panic and anxiety. The effects of caffeine withdrawal—headaches and irritability—may last as long as a week. Nicotine withdrawal can be much more intense. You need to plan carefully to quit smoking by consulting one of the many books available on the subject, or by checking with your health-care professional.

Alcohol

One mythical sleep enhancer is alcohol. You might think of a hot toddy or a nightcap before retiring as relaxing. And it can be—at first. But alcohol taken in larger amounts before bedtime significantly disturbs your ability to maintain sleep. It also contributes to early morning awakening. Some individuals find that even smaller amounts of alcohol have a damaging effect on their sleep. If you are drinking heavily before bedtime in order to numb yourself to sleep or in an attempt to avoid obsessional thinking, you'll find that alcohol only makes matters worse. This has to do with alcohol's disruption of your natural sleep cycles. Researchers have demonstrated that alcohol initially decreases wakefulness, but—as it leaves your body—increases wakefulness in the last half of the night. You may fall asleep quickly, but you'll experience restlessness and fitful sleep later on in the night. The idea is not to use alcohol to sedate yourself to sleep.

Mealtimes

Mealtimes can be scheduled to reprogram your body to feel sleepy. Eat at regular times, and you will get into a routine that can help signal sleep time. If you eat a heavy meal before bedtime, you may find it difficult to relax enough to go to sleep, since your digestive system has to work overtime. For this reason, you'll want to have dinner at least three or four hours before retiring. Space out your other meals at regular intervals, leaving enough time for you to be hungry for an early dinner. If you need a snack before bedtime, drink warm milk or have one of the other foods suggested on the following pages.

Past studies have demonstrated the beneficial effects of L-tryptophan, an amino acid found in such common foods as meat, dairy products, beans, and leafy green vegetables. Before 1989, supplemental doses of L-tryptophan were advised for those suffering from insomnia. The thought was that the amount of L-tryptophan found in common foods was too small to have a significant effect on your sleep. However, the FDA removed L-tryptophan from the market after it was found to contain toxic contaminants from the manufacturing process. Subsequent studies indicate that large amounts of L-tryptophan taken separately can still pose serious health hazards. Since no one is known to have suffered from an old-fashioned glass of warm milk, it may be best to trust mom's advice and return to this natural source of the drug. Consult a doctor for the latest findings before partaking of any L-tryptophan supplements.

L-tryptophan-rich foods eaten before bed can help promote restful sleep, such as turkey, milk, tuna, eggs, fish, almonds, bananas, or peanut butter. And *ice cream*!

A Woman's Guide to Sleep by Joyce Walsleben, Ph.D, and Rita Baron Faust contains great tips for sleep. In their diet section, the authors suggest three sleep-inducing snacks:

Night News Munch
4–5 whole-grain crackers
1–2 ounces sliced turkey, cheese, or leftover tuna salad
8 ounces nonfat or 1 percent milk

Breakfast at Bedtime
1 sliced banana
1 cup high-fiber cold cereal
6 ounces nonfat or 1 percent milk
1 teaspoon ground soy nuts, optional

Sleeper Smoothie
1 sliced banana
1–2 teaspoons banana extract
½ cup fresh strawberries
artificial sweetener to taste
9½ ounces (½ cake) silken tofu
¼ cup soy milk
6 ounces nonfat or 1 percent milk

Blend in electric blender until creamy. Add more flavoring extract and milk if needed.

(An important ingredient in the last two recipes is soy, which contains isoflavones, also known as plant estrogens. These are naturally occurring compounds found in soy products and red clover, and may be especially helpful for sleep disrupted by hot flashes. For more on this, see chapter 14 on complementary and alternative approaches.)

Licensed acupuncturist Brenda Beeley writes in *Menopause and Osteoporosis* that calcium (500 mg) and magnesium (250 mg) taken before bed can act as natural tranquilizers. The B-complex vitamins also help calm nerves and restore the adrenals. Calcium-rich foods are dark green leafy vegetables, tofu and tempeh, soy products, miso, almonds, seaweeds, salmon, sardines, and figs. Conversely, calcium "robbers" are smoking, coffee/caffeine, sugar, alcohol, salt, high-protein diet (especially red meat), phosphates, carbonated drinks, diuretics, and aluminum-containing antacids.

Rigid weight loss plans can have an understandably negative effect on sleep quality. You may wake up in the middle of the night with hunger pangs. Try to space out your caloric intake throughout the day, so that you are able to consume some calories before bedtime to get you through the night.

Exercise

Exercise can be a key to helping you sleep better. Regular exercise has many benefits, psychological and emotional as well as physical. True, it can be hard to overcome inertia and get yourself started. But the good news is that just a little exercise—taking a walk or gardening—can help alleviate depression, raise self-esteem, and promote a sense of well-being, all of which can benefit sleep. Regular exercise is habit forming and a fine replacement for the many less-healthy addictions you may struggle to break. Studies of the effects of an aerobic exercise regimen show that exercisers tend to have lower blood pressure, anxiety, and muscle tension, and are able to cope better with stress than nonexercisers. Studies also show that even simple regular exercise—stretching, strengthening, and gentle movements—helps people sleep better compared to those who are completely sedentary. This may be because exercise promotes the release of certain chemical substances in your brain—neurotransmitters thought to be connected to feelings of well-being and satisfaction.

But the key word here is *regular.* Sporadic bursts of strenuous exercise may prove more painful than helpful. There is one other caveat about exercise: *avoid* exercise just before bedtime. Moderate or strenuous exercise has an initially arousing effect, making it difficult for you to relax. Many studies suggest that the best time of day to exercise is in the afternoon or early evening. Leave yourself about three hours between exercising and bedtime. That gives your body time to enjoy an athletic high, unwind slowly, and begin to want to rest.

The American College of Sports Medicine recommends that you spend twenty to sixty minutes, three to five days per week, doing some sort of aerobic exercise. Examples of appropriate aerobic exercises are running, brisk walking, swimming, cycling, rowing, aerobic dancing, cross-country skiing, and rope skipping. If you are over forty-five or have heart disease risk factors, it's best to consult your health-care professional before embarking on any exercise program.

Other types of exercise you may want to explore are those that promote strength building, such as weight training, yoga, and tai chi. Yoga, for example, uses stretching and deep breathing while focusing on meditative techniques. The repeated movements of tai chi encourage focus and balance. Lifting weights has proven to be especially helpful to women facing bone density loss in midlife. All of these types of exercises have an indirect effect on your sleep by encouraging your general sense of well-being.

Time Scheduling and Other Behaviors

The importance of regular mealtimes has already been mentioned in the section on Diet Do's and Don'ts. It bears repeating, however, that following a *regular schedule* can help "cue" your sleep urge. In an attempt to compensate for poor sleep, many insomniacs go to

bed too early and try to force sleep. Or, they sleep late in the morning and take long naps. It is important for you to go to bed *only*
when you are sleepy. In addition, make yourself get up at the same
time every morning—weekday and weekend, if you can. And, as
you'll see below, it's essential that you skip naps. In general, insomniacs need to reregulate their timing systems and synchronize their
internal clocks as closely as possible with the twenty-four-hour day.
For more information about biological rhythms, see chapter 7.

Following a routine pre-bed ritual can help cue sleepiness,
such as turning on a certain light in the bedroom at the same
time each night. You might leave a not-too-exciting book or novel
on your bedside table and read a chapter each night. Or re-
arrange your pillows in a certain way. One friend reported that all
she had to do was pick up this book or any other on sleep and she
could feel her eyelids begin to droop. She surmised that it was
her inner self reassuring her that there was "help out there," and
that was all she needed to relax.

Avoid arousing, nonsleep enhancing activities just before bedtime, such as eating, watching an exciting movie, or anything else
that gets your juices flowing. An exception is sexual activity, which
tends to be relaxing for most people. If, however, you are a person
who finds sex unsatisfying and worrisome (for example, a person
who is impotent or nonorgasmic) you may want to consult a health-
care professional for counseling. Emotional distress in the form
of sexual difficulty can be a major contributor to insomnia, and
should not be overlooked when trying to unravel a sleep problem.

To learn more about manipulating your daily activities to enhance sleep cues, see chapter 5, "Reconditioning Insomnia."

Naps

As a general rule, insomniacs would be wise to avoid napping.
Naps only reinforce your poor nighttime sleep routine. There are
some exceptions, however.

Much of napping's benefit depends on the time of day the nap is taken. This relates to your body's circadian rhythm, which varies greatly with each individual. (Please refer to chapter 7 for more information on circadian rhythms.) A ten-minute to twenty-minute nap may refresh your midday, without affecting your nighttime sleepiness. You might experiment to find the best time for such a catnap, if you find it helpful. If you work odd hours, you may also find yourself in need of a refresher or a break between different activities. But in general, *naps should not be used to replace lost and broken sleep.* Studies show that napping cannot substitute for a solid night of good sleep.

Don't let yourself use naps to avoid certain tasks or to compensate for feelings of despair and depression. If you have an underlying problem such as depression, naps can often be draining instead of refreshing. They also do little to help solve your problem—the depression, the unpleasant tasks, or the insomnia. Work on staying up during the day, and you'll be more likely to sleep during the night.

On the pro side of napping, if you feel yourself getting anxious about not getting enough sleep at night, a short nap may be reassuring. James Kiley, Ph.D., Director of the National Center on Sleep Disorders Research comments on napping and the elderly. In the National Institute of Health's Word on Health issue (June 1998), he says that "With older people in particular, napping is a good practice. Because their sleep is fragmented and they get less of it at night, they typically make up for it with naps during the day." He goes on to say that napping can increase productivity and help restore your ability to think.

Environmental Factors to Consider

Noise

If you suspect that you are particularly sensitive to noise, take stock of the noise situation in your bedroom. Researchers have found that sensitivity to noise increases as people age, and that women seem more sensitive to noise than men. Don't overlook the obvious such as a cranky cat meowing about or an old sick dog. You may need to make other arrangements for them. If you have noisy neighbors or live near an airport or freeway—and moving is not an option—look into soundproofing your bedroom. This can be done by adding insulation or special building materials to the walls. Healthy, satisfying sleep is worth the added expense. A cheaper alternative is to experiment with various types of "white noise," such as fans, air conditioners, or recordings of natural sounds such as rain or ocean waves. You can also inquire about the latest in earplugs, such as the cylindrical foam earplugs available in drugstores. Check out www.dapworld.com where you can purchase sleep products such as earplugs and foam-lined eye masks with aromatherapy lotions.

Light and Safety

If you are disturbed or awakened by too much light in your bedroom, experiment with different types of eye shades, window shades, and light-blocking curtains. If the blackness of the night makes you uneasy, buy a nightlight and plug it in where you can see it easily. But notice if you wake up throughout the night to check out the nightlight. These micro-awakenings can be enough to disturb your sleep.

If you are feeling unsafe in your location, consider some devices that might make you feel safer and thus more inclined to sleep fully. Make sure there is a cell phone or regular phone within reach of your bed. Take the time to secure your doors and windows. Check to see if the smoke detector works. If you sense your sleep will continue to be eroded by an underlying safety fear, consider investing in a burglar alarm system connected to the local police.

Don't forget to appraise the quality of your mattress. Is it too firm or too soft? I once complained of annoying hip pain for weeks until I slept on a very firm mattress and the pain disappeared. If you have another person sleeping with you, is your bed big enough? Experiment with different kinds of pillows for your head and/or body. Back pain can be alleviated with the right pillow tucked under or between your knees.

Room Temperature

Another researcher, Dr. Peter Hauri, found that when room temperature rises above seventy-five degrees Fahrenheit, people wake up more often, experience more restless sleep and less dreaming sleep, and sleep less deeply. The opposite extreme also presents problems: if the room is too cold, you're probably unable to fall asleep. Optimum temperatures range somewhere between sixty-five and seventy degrees Fahrenheit.

Clocks

Get rid of preset hourly watch beepers or chimers if they disturb your sleep even in the slightest amount. While some people can tune out external noise such as a chiming clock, others may find that the hourly gong only reinforces their obsessional characteristics by reminding them of each passing hour. If you find yourself counting each hour that passes and anticipating the next chime, indicating another sleepless hour, then turn it off.

Bedmate

The presence or absence of a bed partner can be a significant sleep factor. A restless bedmate or a loud snorer is likely to disturb your sleep. You might try earplugs, a mattress specially designed to minimize bouncing, or even separate beds if the problem warrants. Of course, you'll want to help your bedmate solve his or her sleep problems; remember, snoring can denote a more profound medical problem. At the other extreme, if you are accustomed to your bedmate, you may find it hard to sleep well alone.

Sound Therapy

Dr. Jeffrey Thompson is an internationally recognized expert in the field of brain wave frequencies incorporated into musical soundtracks. His work is based on the principles of EEG neuro-feedback, or monitoring the types of frequency waves emitted by the human brain. The theory is that a person can alter states of consciousness from alert to relaxation for optimal mind/body healing. Dr. Thompson says that since the human body is more than 70 percent water, and since sound travels five times more efficiently through the water than air, sound frequency pulse waves played directly into the body have a profound effect on the body's nervous system. The pulse waves, embedded in musical soundtracks, are transmitted into the brain and down through the spinal cord, especially in the hypocampus/limbic system of the brain, where emotions are processed. Far-reaching possibilities are inherent in using this type of vibrational technology in the areas of healing and stress reduction and relaxation.

Dr. Thompson's series of *Brainwave Suites* produced by The Relaxation Company blend subtle pulses of sound into a musical soundtrack that stimulates your brain to produce natural wave patterns that match the state of mind you desire. For example, the company produced a CD devoted to letting go of stress and promoting rejuvenating sleep by encouraging delta waves, the deepest state of sleep. Check it out at www.therelaxationcompany.com.

Using a Sleep Diary

You can use the following sleep diary to monitor your sleep progress. Daily and diligent use of a sleep diary can provide you with an overall picture of your sleep patterns and habits. Do not be concerned with answering the questions perfectly. For example, estimate the number of minutes it generally took you to fall asleep, rather than obsess about getting all the minutes recorded exactly right.

This tool is intended to reinforce positive behaviors by providing you with a subjective assessment. On the bottom of each day's entry record any information that you feel affects the quality of sleep, such as a particular relaxation exercise you are trying, or the amount of exercise you got that day. Don't forget to include the amount of medications, alcohol, or nicotine used, if applicable.

The NSF has graciously agreed to provide us with its sleep diary. It takes only a few minutes each day to complete. NSF suggests you keep it in one convenient place, such as on your bedside table. Complete the diary for seven consecutive days, or copy it and use it for a longer period of time. Then, look over the diary to see if there are any patterns or practices that may be contributing to your sleep problems. Discuss any sleep problems with your health-care provider; bring the completed sleep diary with you to help you get the most out of your visit.

National Sleep Foundation Sleep Diary

	COMPLETE IN MORNING							COMPLETE AT END OF DAY				
Fill out days 1–4 below and days 5–7 on page 2	I went to bed last night at:	I got out of bed this morning at:	Last night, I fell asleep in: *(Record number of times)*	I woke up during the night: *(Record number of times)*	When I woke up for the day, I felt: *(Check one)*	Last night I slept a total of: *(Record number of hours)*	My sleep was disturbed by: *(List any mental, emotional, physical or environmental factors that affected your sleep, e.g. stress, snoring, physical discomfort, temperature)*	I consumed caffeinated drinks in the: *(e.g. coffee, tea, cola)*	I exercised at least 20 minutes in the:	Approximately 2–3 hours before going to bed, I consumed:	Medication(s) I took during the day: *[List name of medication/drug(s)]*	About 1 hour before going to sleep, I did the following activity: *(List activity, e.g. watch TV, work, read)*
DAY 1 DAY _____ DATE _____	_____ PM/AM	_____ PM/AM	_____ Minutes	_____ Times	□ Refreshed □ Somewhat refreshed □ Fatigued	_____ Hours		□ Morning □ Afternoon □ Within several hours before going to bed □ Not applicable	□ Morning □ Afternoon □ Within several hours before going to bed □ Not applicable	□ Alcohol □ A heavy meal □ Not applicable		
DAY 2 DAY _____ DATE _____	_____ PM/AM	_____ PM/AM	_____ Minutes	_____ Times	□ Refreshed □ Somewhat refreshed □ Fatigued	_____ Hours		□ Morning □ Afternoon □ Within several hours before going to bed □ Not applicable	□ Morning □ Afternoon □ Within several hours before going to bed □ Not applicable	□ Alcohol □ A heavy meal □ Not applicable		
DAY 3 DAY _____ DATE _____	_____ PM/AM	_____ PM/AM	_____ Minutes	_____ Times	□ Refreshed □ Somewhat refreshed □ Fatigued	_____ Hours		□ Morning □ Afternoon □ Within several hours before going to bed □ Not applicable	□ Morning □ Afternoon □ Within several hours before going to bed □ Not applicable	□ Alcohol □ A heavy meal □ Not applicable		
DAY 4 DAY _____ DATE _____	_____ PM/AM	_____ PM/AM	_____ Minutes	_____ Times	□ Refreshed □ Somewhat refreshed □ Fatigued	_____ Hours		□ Morning □ Afternoon □ Within several hours before going to bed □ Not applicable	□ Morning □ Afternoon □ Within several hours before going to bed □ Not applicable	□ Alcohol □ A heavy meal □ Not applicable		

National Sleep Foundation Sleep Diary

Fill out days 5–7 below	COMPLETE IN MORNING							COMPLETE AT END OF DAY				
	I went to bed last night at:	I got out of bed this morning at:	Last night, I fell asleep in:	I woke up during the night: *(Record number of times)*	When I woke up for the day, I felt: *(Check one)*	Last night I slept a total of: *(Record number of hours)*	My sleep was disturbed by: *(List any mental, emotional, physical or environmental factors that affected your sleep; e.g. stress, snoring, physical discomfort, temperature)*	I consumed caffeinated drinks in the: *(e.g. coffee, tea, cola)*	I exercised at least 20 minutes in the:	Approximately 2–3 hours before going to bed, I consumed:	Medication(s) I took during the day: *[List name of medication/drug(s)]*	About 1 hour before going to sleep, I did the following activity: *(List activity, e.g. watch TV, work, read)*
DAY 5 DAY ——— DATE ———	——— PM/AM	——— PM/AM	——— Minutes	——— Times	☐ Refreshed ☐ Somewhat refreshed ☐ Fatigued	——— Hours		☐ Morning ☐ Afternoon ☐ Within several hours before going to bed ☐ Not applicable	☐ Morning ☐ Afternoon ☐ Within several hours before going to bed ☐ Not applicable	☐ Alcohol ☐ A heavy meal ☐ Not applicable		
DAY 6 DAY ——— DATE ———	——— PM/AM	——— PM/AM	——— Minutes	——— Times	☐ Refreshed ☐ Somewhat refreshed ☐ Fatigued	——— Hours		☐ Morning ☐ Afternoon ☐ Within several hours before going to bed ☐ Not applicable	☐ Morning ☐ Afternoon ☐ Within several hours before going to bed ☐ Not applicable	☐ Alcohol ☐ A heavy meal ☐ Not applicable		
DAY 7 DAY ——— DATE ———	——— PM/AM	——— PM/AM	——— Minutes	——— Times	☐ Refreshed ☐ Somewhat refreshed ☐ Fatigued	——— Hours		☐ Morning ☐ Afternoon ☐ Within several hours before going to bed ☐ Not applicable	☐ Morning ☐ Afternoon ☐ Within several hours before going to bed ☐ Not applicable	☐ Alcohol ☐ A heavy meal ☐ Not applicable		

3

Relaxation for Sleep

Whether you suffer from transient or persistent insomnia, you'll not want to overlook the benefits of regular and *intentional* relaxation. Many people overlook this basic physical need to relax, assuming that they already know about it. They may unwittingly choose to live with a high level of physical and emotional tension, which builds up over time.

There are two simple and compelling reasons to practice relaxation. First, the experience of insomnia is itself a stress factor. It reduces your ability to function, to cope, and to feel good—both mentally and physically. If you can't function, you feel useless. If you can't cope, then stressors begin to pile up. Second, you tense your muscles in response to these negative feelings and behaviors. You grit your teeth in anticipation of sleeplessness. This increases your body's overall tension level, which only makes your nightly battle worse.

The first step toward healthy sleep is to realize that physical tension and mental anxiety can make coping more difficult. It's a vicious circle—but you can break it by learning to manage the tension in your life. You can learn to identify stress in your body and control its interplay with your sleeplessness.

This chapter presents an array of relaxation exercises, adapted here to suit the special need of insomniacs. The exercises you see in this chapter can be used in preparation for bedtime, during sleep onset, and throughout the course of the night should you happen to awaken. The first three exercises, Deep Breathing, Progressive Muscle Relaxation (PMR), and Autogenic Training (AT), form a solid basis of any relaxation endeavor, and can be customized to suit your particular needs and tastes anywhere, anytime. Following these sections, you will find descriptions of ways to assist relaxation by using biofeedback or neurofeedback, best learned with the help of a health-care practitioner.

All of these exercises can be done separately or in combination with each other. If you are unfamiliar with using relaxation techniques to reduce tension and anxiety, begin by trying each exercise separately. Give yourself at least one week of daily practice of each, preferably twice a day, before you begin mixing and matching the techniques. After you become comfortable with the feel of each exercise, you can begin to experiment with shortening or lengthening each exercise to suit your needs.

Be sure to practice your technique selection at least once during the day. You will find that with systematic practice, these exercises can be especially effective in counteracting the buildup of anxiety throughout the day. That's a big step toward eliminating a primary cause of insomnia.

Deep Breathing

It's easy to forget about the soothing qualities of fresh air in your lungs. If you've been tense all day following a hectic schedule, and your first chance to relax comes in the evening hour just before bed, it's no wonder that relaxing sufficiently to fall asleep is a problem. Deep breathing—also known as "diaphragmatic breathing" or "abdominal breathing"—is one of the most practical ways to relax quickly and effectively. In addition, it helps to counteract oxygen-starved and stressed out bodies by expanding the bottom half of the lung. As you inhale, gently pushing your stomach muscles out, up, and away from your body, you are forcing air into the lower halves of your lungs. Typical breathing is usually rapid and shallow, causing only a partial exchange of oxygen with carbon dioxide. When an insufficient amount of fresh air reaches your lungs, your blood is not cleansed of the waste-carrying carbon dioxide circulated by the blood that contributes to undernourished tissue and organs, depression, anxiety, and fatigue. When practiced regularly, deep breathing counteracts these effects and sets off a chain reaction of physical and emotional well-being.

Deep breathing can be practiced anywhere—in the office, riding the bus, driving, at home, before bedtime—while sitting, standing, or lying down. But to become comfortable with the technique, it is recommended that you first focus your attention on abdominal breathing while lying on your back. Once it has become automatic for you, it will take only seconds to use it anywhere, anytime, to help relieve tension.

You'll soon find that deep breathing combines nicely with the other forms of relaxation found in this chapter. Before you flip the pages to those, however, focus your attention on deep breathing. It is the foundation on which relaxed bodies are built.

Deep Breathing on Your Back

Lying on your back, place one hand on your chest, and the other on your abdomen. Uncross your legs, allowing them to be spread comfortably apart or bent at the knees with both feet flat on the floor.

a. Inhale slowly through your nostrils.
b. Feel the breath move through your chest, raising that hand slightly. As the breath reaches your stomach, push your

abdomen upward toward the ceiling, while completing your inhalation. Allow the hand on your abdomen to rise slightly higher than the hand on your chest.

c. Hold for a second, then reverse the process, allowing the breath to pass back out through chest and nostrils. As you exhale, feel your muscles let go of tension. Allow your jaw to unclench as you exhale.

d. Focus on this breathing process twice each day, for a period of ten to twenty minutes each time. Your body will tell you when you are comfortable with this breathing, and you will soon be able to apply it automatically when your body tenses up.

Deep Breathing on Your Stomach

This is an excellent exercise for practicing abdominal breathing, especially if you have difficulty feeling the movement of the diaphragm while breathing in a sitting or lying position.

a. Lie on your stomach, placing your legs a comfortable distance apart with toes pointed outward. Fold arms in front of your body, resting hands on biceps. Position arms so that the chest does not touch the floor.

b. As you inhale, feel the diaphragmatic motion while in this position.

Points to remember about deep breathing:

1. Deep breathing can serve as a preventative tool to help you guard against the buildup of tension levels. Monitor yourself throughout the day. At the first signs of stress, take a few moments to do five or six good, deep breaths. You can do this anywhere, anytime, sitting or standing. Simply close your eyes and focus on your breathing, slowing it and

deepening it. Do this as many times during the day as necessary to help calm yourself. With persistence, you'll begin to notice the accumulation of calm by the end of the day, rather than the buildup of stress.

2. Develop the ability to "concentrate passively" on your deep breathing. The concept of passive concentration or passive volition is well known in Eastern philosophy, but less understood in Western culture where striving for perfection is emphasized. Passive concentration enables you to focus on what you are doing, but in such a way that you are comfortably observing your actions, almost as if you were watching yourself from afar. In other words, you allow yourself to breathe deeply rather than forcing yourself to do it perfectly. A common problem with ambitious achievers who are attempting to relax is that they expect themselves to relax perfectly when they command it. They then get frustrated when stray thoughts of business or pleasure interrupt their task. They try to force the thoughts away. They work too hard! If you feel you have to do the deep breathing and other exercises in this chapter "just right" in order for you to be successful, then consider that you are working against yourself and your goal here—relaxation. Repeat to yourself over and over, "I am *allowing* myself to relax." See your extraneous thoughts pass through your mind. Eventually they will cease to clutter your mind, but let that time naturally evolve by itself. Permit yourself *not* to do it just right all the time.

On-the-Spot Deep Breathing

Whenever you feel troubling thoughts creep into your consciousness, either in the hours before bed or as your head hits the pillow, you probably feel your muscles tensing. Common areas for tension are the abdomen, shoulders, and jaw. *As soon as you feel your muscles tensing,* repeat these simple deep breathing steps:

1. Inhale slowly, pushing the stomach muscles *out*. If it helps, put your hand on your stomach to feel the muscles extending outward as you inhale. This helps elongate your lower lung area, which in turn gets you more breath for the effort, and fills your lungs with healing, soothing oxygen.
2. Exhale slowly, feeling your stomach muscles collapse, and the rest of your muscles melt into the bed.
3. As you exhale, repeat a generic calming phrase to yourself, such as: "I am calm," "One," or "Peace." You might prefer a calming phrase specific to sleep inducement, such as: "Sleep is coming on," "I can sleep now," "Sleep is replacing my worries."

Breath-Counting Meditation

Breath counting is a popular combination of deep breathing and meditation. Instead of using mantras, which seem strange to some people, breath counting simply involves numbering each breath. In this way, you narrow the focus of your attention on the process of relaxation and away from daily distractions.

1. Go to a quiet place and center your eyes or gaze at a spot in the room or on the wall.
2. Begin deep breathing. As you exhale, say silently to yourself, "one." Continue to breathe in and out, saying "one" each time you exhale.
3. When thoughts distract you from your breathing, allow yourself to let go of them and return to saying "one." Practice breath counting for at least ten to twenty minutes at a time.

4. A variation on breath counting is to continue counting each exhalation from one to four: Inhale . . . exhale, saying "one." Inhale . . . exhale, saying "two." And so forth. When you reach "four," start over again.

For more about meditation techniques, please see the meditation section in chapter 4.

Progressive Muscle Relaxation

Tense people, especially when preoccupied with whether they will go to sleep or not, often have tense muscles. If you find yourself lying in bed and obsessing about a particularly tense muscle, then you may find it harder and harder to relax. Have you ever felt a leg muscle cramp up when you thought about it, even though you tried hard not to? The harder you tried, the more tense you became.

Progressive Muscle Relaxation (PMR) was developed forty years ago by a doctor named Edmund Jacobson. He wanted his patients to be able to differentiate clearly between a tensed and a relaxed muscle, and so he developed a process that intentionally contracted and released the tensed muscle. To do PMR, all you have to do is focus on the cramped muscle, tense it gently, and then relax it. You can relax. You can relax your whole body this way. You begin with a muscle group at one end of your body, for example your toes or facial muscles, and systematically work up or down through as many muscle groups as you choose.

This exercise can be a very effective way to learn about the *amount* of muscle tension you carry in your body. It will also help you feel the sharp contrast between tensed muscles and relaxed muscles. It is easy to walk around with clenched teeth or fists all day and not even realize it. Until, that is, the end of the day when you have a tension headache or a sore shoulder. Sometimes when you think you have relaxed your muscles, they may still be contracted tightly, causing muscle fatigue, poor circulation, cramping, and stiffness. Ease into this exercise slowly and don't strain yourself.

You will be focusing on four major groups of muscles in the body:

- Hands, forearms, and biceps
- Thighs, buttocks, calves, and feet
- Chest, stomach, and lower back
- Head, face, throat, neck, and shoulders. Facial muscles include forehead, cheeks, nose, eyes, jaws, lips, and tongue.

Once you have read through the description below, try to spend at least twenty minutes per day on each muscle group. It is usually helpful to follow along with a tape or CD at first. You can buy a premade tape or CD at many bookstores Web sites such as mindbyte.net, or sleep labs, or make one yourself using the script below.

Dr. Hauri, acclaimed sleep researcher and writer, in *No More Sleepless Nights* suggests practicing PMR separately from sleep time to be sure you notice what is happening with your body, and you're not just falling asleep. Then when you feel comfortable with the technique, eliminate the tensing phase. He suggests that this technique can be a very effective sleep inducer by simply making mental contact with each muscle group and letting the muscles experience the same degree of relaxation that comes over them naturally after tensing.

Begin PMR by lying down or sitting in a comfortable chair with your head supported. Take several deep breaths, releasing each breath slowly. This deep and natural breathing is your cue to begin your relaxation session.

1. Focus on the first group of muscles—your right hand, arm, and biceps. Make a fist, clenching as hard as you can. Hold that tension, feeling it creep up your arm toward your

shoulder. Hold it until you begin to feel a gentle cramping
or burning sensation. You may notice your muscles quiver
slightly.

2. Now relax, feeling the muscles go limp. Feel the warming
blood flow through your arm into your hand and fingers.
Notice the contrast between what it felt like when it was
tense, and what it feels like now when it is relaxed.

3. Repeat this twice. Remember to pay attention to your
breathing as you tense and relax. Does your breathing begin
to get shallow? Make sure you are not unconsciously holding your breath.

4. Now notice how the right arm and hand feel compared to
the left arm and hand. Move to your left hand, arm, and
biceps to repeat the exercise three times.

After a few days of this muscle group, move on to the second
group: thighs, buttocks, calves, and feet. Repeat the same procedure as above, alternating sides of your body.

1. Focus on your right foot and calf. Tighten them as hard as
you can. You can either pull your foot upward, or stretch
your foot outward by pointing your toe. Hold the tension,
feeling it creep up your leg toward your torso. Hold the
tension till you begin to feel a slight cramping, burning
sensation.

2. Now relax, feeling the muscles go limp. Feel the warming
blood flow through your calf and foot. Notice the contrast
between what your muscles felt like when you were tense,
and what they feel like now that you are relaxed.

3. Repeat this procedure twice. Remember to pay attention
to your breathing as you tense and relax. Does your breathing begin to get shallow? Make sure you are not unconsciously holding your breath.

4. Now notice how the right calf and foot feel in comparison to the left calf and foot. Focus on your left calf and foot and repeat the exercise three times.
5. Now focus on your right leg again. Tense your thigh and buttocks as you tense your foot and calf. Tense as hard as you can, until you begin to feel a slight cramping and burning sensation.
6. Now relax, feeling all the muscles in your right leg go limp. Feel the warming blood flow through your buttocks, thigh, calf, and foot. Notice the contrast between what your leg felt like when it was tense, and what it feels like now when it is relaxed.
7. Repeat this procedure twice. Remember to keep your breathing relaxed and natural. Notice how your right leg feels in comparison to your left leg.
8. Move to your left leg, adding the buttocks and thigh to your left foot and calf. Repeat the exercise three times.

Spend the next two to three days of your practice on group three: chest, stomach, and lower back. Remember to breathe deeply and exhale slowly as you release the tension in your stomach. If you have lower back pain, proceed cautiously with the tensing of your back muscles. Contract the muscles as much as you can, but do not strain or overdo it.

1. Focus on your chest, stomach, and lower back. Tense those areas, lightly pushing your lower back into the bed or chair as you contract your abdominal muscles and shrug your shoulders. Hold the tension until you begin to feel a slight cramping, burning sensation.
2. Now relax, feeling the muscles go limp. Feel the warming blood flow through your lower back, stomach, and chest. Notice the contrast between what it felt like when these

areas were tense, and what it feels like now when they are relaxed.
3. Repeat this procedure twice. Remember to keep your breathing relaxed and natural.

Now move on to the next muscle group: the head, face neck, and shoulder muscles. Pay special attention to the facial muscles. They are extremely sensitive to stress and anxiety. Your jaw muscles are so powerful that you can be tensing them all day without realizing it. You can use the following script:

Facial PMR

Turning attention to your head, wrinkle your forehead as tight as you can. Lift your eyebrows as high as they will go. Now relax and smooth it out. Let yourself imagine your entire forehead and scalp becoming smooth and at rest. Repeat.

Now frown and notice the strain spreading throughout your forehead. Where else is it tense? Your jaw? Your neck? Let go. Allow your brow to become smooth again. Close your eyes now, squint them tighter. Scan for tension. Relax your eyes. Let them remain closed gently and comfortably.

Now clench your jaw. Bite hard. Notice the tension throughout your jaw. This muscle is very powerful, and you may not be aware of the amount of tension it can hold. Relax your jaw. When the jaw is relaxed, your lips will be slightly parted. Let yourself really appreciate the contrast between tension and relaxation. Think of your jaw as two unconnected halves—top and bottom untouching.

Now press your tongue against the roof of your mouth. Push it hard against the top. Feel the ache in the back of your mouth and the tip of your tongue. Relax. Press your lips now, purse them into an "O." Relax your lips. Notice that your forehead, scalp, eyes, jaw, tongue, and lips are all relaxed.

A Variation on PMR: Differential Relaxation

Differential relaxation simply means tensing and relaxing as you would with PMR, but doing it with diagonal muscle groups at the same time. For example, starting with muscle groups one and two, tense your right arm and hand and left leg and foot at the same time. Also release simultaneously. As you tense, pay attention to the sides of your body you are not tensing. (Left arm, hand and right leg, foot.) This may take some practice.

The purpose of differential relaxation is to introduce you to a slightly more complex exercise that more closely resembles your daily activity. A common example is that when you drive, you often unconsciously clench your teeth and jaw in response to traffic or the normal wear and tear of driving. This locks in needless additional tension. Of course, you don't want to relax *all* of your body while driving. You need to keep your leg and foot tense and alert on the accelerator pedal. Differential relaxation teaches you how to tense one part of the body, while keeping the other relaxed.

As you practice this exercise, pay attention to the feeling of tension on the tense side, *and* the feeling of relaxation on the relaxed side. By doing so simultaneously, you are encouraging your brain to develop a multiple capacity for relaxing. In other words, you are learning to be alert and relaxed at the same time. This exercise will help you learn to easily adapt other forms of relaxation to your everyday activity.

Remember not to rush through each muscle group while practicing differential relaxation of PMR. Allow yourself the luxury of a sufficient amount of time per muscle group.

You may also find it useful to repeat the following sentences out loud while releasing your muscle tension:

> Let go of the tension.
> Relax and smooth out the muscles.
> Let the tension dissolve away.
> Let go more and more.

Autogenic Training

In the 1930s, two physicians named Johannes Schultz and Wolf-gang Luthe found that they could help their patients reduce fatigue by teaching them to self-generate feelings of heaviness with the muscles. As with PMR, Autogenic Training (AT) works on the principle that the brain can give messages of warmth and relaxation to the blood vessels, which in turn relax your muscles, and even internal organs.

Sometimes the process of contracting/releasing is more stimulating than relaxing, and you might find that you prefer a more passive exercise. Insomniacs are renowned for their high anxiety levels, and sometimes a passive activity distracts a highly anxious person more effectively than a physical activity. In addition, studies show that AT encourages the actual flow of blood to the extremities. Stressed-out people have a tendency toward poorer circulation. AT can help to reverse this, allowing the hands and feet to be warmer because of the better blood flow. This helps you feel more overall relaxation. It also demonstrates your brain's tremendous control over your body. After you feel your body responding to the standard AT phrases below, you can customize the phrases to suit your imagination. For example, you might warm your hands and then move them to a sore muscle, as if your hands were a hot-water bottle. Or, move your warmed hands to your forehead. Imagine that the added warmth is melting away all obsessive and distracting thoughts.

You will focus on the same four muscle groups as you did with PMR:

- Hands and arms
- Thighs, buttocks, legs, and feet
- Chest, stomach, and lower back
- Head, face, throat, neck, and shoulders

Spend at least twenty minutes per day on each muscle group, and approximately one full week of practice for each group. Usually it is helpful to follow along with a tape at first. You can buy a pre-made tape, or make one yourself using the script below (adapted from *The Relaxation Training Program* by Thomas Budzinski).

Begin AT by lying down or sitting in a comfortable chair with your head supported. Take several deep breaths, releasing each breath slowly. This deep and natural breathing is your cue to begin your relaxation session.

1. Focus on the first muscle group, beginning with your right hand and arm. Lay your arm flat on an armrest, a tabletop, or your lap. Your aim is to become intensely aware of the muscles and fibers in your arm and hand—and then let them go. Feel the warmth and weight as you repeat the phrases:

   My right hand is heavy.
   My right hand is heavy and warm.
   My right hand is letting go.

   My right arm is heavy.
   My right arm is heavy and warm.
   My right arm is letting go.

   Repeat each set of phrases twice, then move to your left hand and arm. Feel your arm float on its own as you allow your blood to flow from your shoulder through your elbow to the tips of your fingers.

   My left hand is heavy.
   My left hand is heavy and warm.
   My left hand is letting go.

   My left arm is heavy.
   My left arm is heavy and warm.
   My left arm is letting go.

2. After several days on the first group, move on to the second group: your feet, calves, thighs, and buttocks. Repeat the same phrases as above, inserting the words for the desired body group. For example, "My right leg is heavy," and so on. My right thigh is heavy and warm. My chest is letting go, and so on.

Next, move to group three: stomach, chest, and lower back.

Then focus on group four: shoulders, neck throat, face, and head. Repeat the phrases to yourself, focusing first on your shoulders, then neck and throat, then head and face.

As you become comfortable and adept at AT phrases, you can add additional instructions, such as "My right arm is loose and limp." Remember to check your breathing periodically to make sure you are breathing by imagining the blood flowing to your extremities as you exhale.

It is helpful and natural to incorporate imagery into your AT work. Some examples might be to imagine the sun warming your hands as you repeat the phrases, or that you are lying in a warm bath, or any other scene that comes to mind and represents heaviness and warmth.

These additional sentences from the *Relaxation and Stress Reduction Workbook* may be used while you repeat the autogenic phrases, or you may repeat them to yourself at the end of your session.

> I feel quiet.
> My whole body feels quiet, heavy, comfortable, and relaxed.
> My mind is quiet.
> I withdraw my thoughts from the surroundings and I feel serene and still.
> My thoughts are turned inward and I am at ease.

Deep within my mind, I can visualize and experience
myself as relaxed and comfortable and still.
I feel an inward quietness.

Remember to adopt an attitude of passive concentration while practicing your AT techniques. This means, do not force yourself to concentrate. Rather, *allow* yourself to focus on the exercises. When extraneous thoughts intrude upon your concentration, simply allow them to pass through your mind. Eventually, with practice, they will become less numerous and intrusive.

Add deep breathing to your repetitions of AT phrases: Make use of the healing properties of oxygen and deep breathing by including deep breathing with your AT phrases. In between sessions of each body section that you are relaxing, pay attention to your breathing. Does your stomach continue to stay relaxed as you repeat the AT phrases? If not, breathe deeply. As you exhale, feel your jaw drop open, and the healing warmth of oxygenated blood rush into each muscle.

Relaxation Aided by Biofeedback

Biofeedback involves the use of instruments to measure muscle tension, blood flow, heart rate, and more. These measurements are indicators of your stress level. For example, if you unknowingly clench your jaw, this tends to increase the muscle tension in your face, neck, and shoulders. If you were hooked up to a biofeedback machine, it would record a high level of muscle contractions in that area, indicating a high level of muscle tension there. Muscle tension levels are typically measured with surface electrodes placed on the forehead area with the help of an electromyogram (EMG). These reveal tension levels in the face, jaw, neck, and shoulders. Biofeedback is not at all painful (or even scary). In fact, it's a very relaxing procedure. You are usually given audio cues (a beeping tone) or visual cues (computer graphs) to tell you how much your muscles are letting go of the tension. As you relax, the graphs diminish and the tone beeps lower and lower.

Sometimes hand temperatures reflect your typical response to stress. Remember the "mood rings" of the 1960s? They operated on this principle. As you become anxious, blood flow is constricted and your extremities can become cold as ice. In biofeedback, electrodes are placed on your fingertips, and you are given information as to when you are becoming warmer, and thus more relaxed.

The biofeedback procedure is intended as a teaching aid. Once you know how it feels to be relaxed and calm according to the instruments, you can transfer that learning to daily activities and nighttime sleep preparation. While most equipment is too cumbersome and expensive to have at home, some simplified versions of biofeedback instruments are available at reasonable prices. These are adequate in reminding you of your tension levels.

There are many modified versions of biofeedback equipment available for at-home use, such as temperature rings, stress dots or cards, or Pulse-O-Meters. As a preventative tool, the ring functions as an early warning system. It has a temperature range of sixty-seven to ninety-four degrees Fahrenheit, with little dots that light up at each point on the range. If you notice your temperature dropping, indicating a possible increase in tension levels, you can use this information as a cue to take note of your situation. Are you feeling anxious? Angry? Or are you simply in a cold room? Once you have this answer, you can apply a therapeutic technique: autogenics and imagery might warm your hands and focus and soothe your mind.

Stress dots also provide you with a general idea of your temperature range. A dot is peeled from a piece of paper and attached to your hand. The dot changes color as your hands change from cool to warm. Stress cards are credit card size and have a temperature indicator warmed by your finger. You can lower a racing heart beat by holding the Pulse-O-Meter in your hand. Your heart rate is displayed in a digital numeric readout. Check the following Web sites for information on where to purchase these handy do-it-yourself relaxation tools: Futurehealth.org or bio-medical.com.

You can incorporate these aids in your nighttime ritual. If you choose to combine deep breathing and meditation as your pre-bed procedure, use the relaxation aids to verify your relaxation response.

4

Meditation, Self-Hypnosis, and Visualization

The time-honored traditions of meditation, self-hypnosis, and visualization are powerful practices for calming the mind and healing the body. These three techniques are grouped because they share common attributes. While each technique varies in its approach, overall they invite you to physically calm your body in preparation for calming and focusing your mind. You pass through to these pleasant feelings of centeredness and peace by first practicing the standard relaxation techniques, such as deep breathing. Your body and mind are prepared for sleep as you learn to filter out extraneous thoughts and focus instead on calming thoughts or images. With practice, you can adapt these techniques to fit your particular sleep needs as well as help reprogram poor sleep habits.

Meditation is described in two ways: the traditional or transcendental form of meditation, which uses the repetition of a mantra, a mind-calming phrase, and Jon Kabat-Zinn's invitation to see meditation as a way to practice mindfulness, or "present moment awareness."

Self-hypnosis employs the use of simple suggestions in a trance state, geared to helping you fall asleep and maintain sleep. Visualization—using images you find pleasant and sleep inducing—is encouraged while you are in a trance or meditative state and can be intentionally shaped to reinforce hypnotic suggestions and posthypnotic cues (which will be discussed later). It takes practice and commitment to excel in any of these techniques, but you don't have to do them perfectly right away to notice the benefits.

Meditation

Meditation is similar in process to the other relaxation exercises presented in this book, in which you minimize distractions and narrow your focus of attention. Traditionally, *transcendental* meditation involves repetition of a "mantra," a word or phrase that you find particularly pleasant and comforting. As you repeat this word over and over, you permit distracting thoughts, sounds, and feelings to pass by uncritically. Without judging them or yourself, you allow these negative thoughts and feelings to fade away, enabling you to return to your mantra. Once you are in a very relaxed state, your consciousness becomes uncluttered and open to suggestion. At this point you are able to give yourself soothing suggestions embodied by the mantra. Whether you choose to practice meditation at some point during the day, or just in preparation for bedtime, remember to pay attention to the following four major components of meditation:

1. Choose a quiet place in which to meditate. Turn down the volume on the answering machine, or turn the phone off altogether. Minimize external distractions wherever possible.
2. Choose a comfortable position that can be maintained for about twenty minutes without causing discomfort. Avoid meditating within two hours of a heavy meal, since digestion interferes with your comfort.

3. It is helpful to select an object to dwell upon: a word or sound repetition, an object or symbol to gaze at or imagine, even a specific feeling or thought. As distracting thoughts enter your mind, you can let them pass while returning to the chosen object of focus.
4. Maintain a passive attitude. When distracting thoughts occur, let go of them, but don't force them to leave. Don't judge yourself or your ability to perform the meditative process. Assume an objective, uncritical stance. Imagine yourself observing yourself repeating your mantra effortlessly and comfortably.

A variation of the meditative technique is the breath-counting exercise described in the deep breathing section in chapter 3.

Meditation as "Mindfulness"

Jon Kabat-Zinn has written extensively about the benefits of meditation in his books *Full Catastrophe Living* and *Wherever You Go There You Are*. He has successfully used his approach to manage stress, pain, and illness at the Stress Reduction Clinic at the University of Massachusetts Medical Center. Mindfulness, or present-moment awareness, is a way of looking deeply into yourself in the spirit of self-inquiry and self-understanding. He calls it "calming the inner busyness." When you begin simply observing your mind, you find there is a great deal of mental and emotional activity going on beneath the surface. These incessant thoughts and feelings can drain away your positive healing energy. Kabat-Zinn says, "What we frequently call formal meditation involves purposefully making a time for stopping all outward activity and cultivating stillness, with no agenda other than being fully present in each moment. Not doing anything. Perhaps such moments of non-doing are the greatest gift one can give oneself."

The following is a recap of the attitudes needed to supply a firm foundation for his mindfulness practice:

1. Be nonjudging. Assume the stance of an impartial witness to your experience.
2. Be patient. Learn to understand and accept the fact that sometimes things must unfold in their own time.
3. Adopt a beginner's mind-set. Avoid already "knowing the answer" and see the richness of the present moment; cultivate a mind that is willing to see everything as if for the first time.
4. Trust yourself. Develop a basic trust in yourself and your feelings. Honor your intuition and inner wisdom.
5. Be nonstriving. Meditation is the ultimate nondoing. It has no goal other than for you to be yourself. Back off from striving for results.
6. Adopt acceptance. See things as they actually are in the present.
7. Let go. Cultivate the attitude of nonattachment.

On this last point, Kabat-Zinn elaborates: "Most of us have experienced times when the mind would just not shut down when we got into bed. This is one of the first signs of elevated stress. At these times we may be unable to free ourselves from certain thoughts because our involvement in them is just too powerful. If we try to force ourselves to sleep, it just makes things worse. So if you can go to sleep, you are already an expert in letting go. Now you just need to practice applying this skill in waking situations as well."

For example, if you are chronically anxious, you apply mindfulness meditation by sitting comfortably in a quiet space, as described above, observing your breathing. You allow the anxiety itself to become the object of your nonjudgmental attention. By moving in close to your fears and observing them as they surface in the form of thoughts, feelings, and physical sensations, you will be in a much better position to know them for what they are. You will be less prone to becoming overwhelmed by them or having to compensate in self-destructive or self-inhibiting ways.

Self-Hypnosis Techniques

The word "hypnosis" often invokes images of things mysterious, but the experience commonly occurs in many unspectacular ways throughout the day. You can probably identify several times in the past week when you lost yourself in concentration, perhaps when driving or watching TV. These states are examples of hypnotic trances, which can be adapted to focus intentionally on an area of difficulty in your life, such as insomnia.

There is a physical difference between sleep and a hypnotic state. In sleep you are not conscious or aware of the world; in hypnosis you are in a calm, peaceable state, but aware. To reinforce this notion, scientists can measure the electrical changes occurring in the brain, called brain waves, during wakefulness and sleep by use of electroencephalographs, or EEGs. For example, your brain emits beta waves while awake and alpha waves while in a state of calm wakefulness. As you drop off to sleep, your brain emits theta waves, and as you sleep deeply, delta waves. You actually move in and out of all of these wave patterns at varying speeds and times throughout the course of the night.

You can use hypnosis to pass through to the unconsciousness of sleep. Your signal for coming out of the trance is when you actually fall asleep. This way you can be assured that you will awaken if you need to. In fact, you are in complete control of your trance state at all times. You can control when to terminate the trance and when to fall peacefully into sleep.

Self-hypnosis uses an induction, or a script, to bring about a trance state. Inductions vary in style and content. Concerning style, you may find that you respond readily to an induction that uses a highly directive, authoritative style, such as: "You will listen to my voice. My voice will help you relax as deeply as possible. I want you to begin to relax now. As you relax deeper and deeper you will respond to the suggestions I give you."

Or, you may prefer a softer, more passive style in your induction, such as: "As you listen to my voice, allow it to help you relax. You can let my voice help you relax as deeply as possible. As you relax more and more deeply, just imagine yourself in a peaceful place. It may be by the ocean or in the mountains. Any place is fine. Imagine how wonderful you feel in this place. Imagine how peaceful you feel there. Now let yourself relax even more deeply, and as you relax, allow yourself to embrace the suggestion that I am about to give you."

You can choose to induce a trance by selecting any of the relaxation exercises described in this book. A popular combination is deep breathing and systematic muscle relaxation. Some people prefer to use the "fixation" method of hypnotic induction, in which attention is drawn to a very narrow point. For example, you can stare into a flickering candle to practice this type of induction. A typical induction might sound like this: "Watch the flame burn and flicker and keep your eyes on the flame and concentrate on it. Watch the flame flicker and keep your eyes on the flame. As you watch the flame burning, your eyes will become heavy, become heavy, and your eyes will grow heavier and heavier . . . and heavier . . . heavier . . . until they close."

You might want to experiment with the different induction approaches and custom-design one to suit your needs. Effective inductions may be quite different from one another, but they must all bring about these results:

- Relaxation of body and mind
- Narrowed focus of attention
- Reduced awareness of external environment and everyday concerns

- Greater internal awareness of sensations
- A trance state

All hypnosis is essentially self-hypnosis. When hypnosis is practiced in a clinic or hospital, a trained therapist guides you through the steps, which you still enact on your own. Sometimes it is useful to begin hypnosis practice under the guidance of a trained clinician who can introduce you to the techniques, guide you in their appropriate uses, and motivate you to follow through on your home practice. Of course, if you already have the motivation, you can use this book as your guide and proceed on your own.

As with the rest of the self-help strategies outlined in this book, self-hypnosis cannot serve as the sole treatment if you suspect you have an underlying medical condition.

Hypnotic Inductions

The following is a general induction adapted for insomniacs. The induction begins with suggestions for overall relaxation and ends with specific posthypnotic sleep instructions. Feel free to insert phrases that customize the induction to suit your particular needs. You can choose to read over an induction to familiarize yourself with it and then repeat it from memory as you relax. Or you may find it easier to make a tape recording of yourself or a friend reading the induction. If you choose to record an induction, here are some suggestions for recording the sample induction that follows.

1. Read the induction aloud several times in order to become familiar and comfortable with its content. When recording, speak slowly and in a monotone, keeping your voice level and your words evenly spaced. You will need to experiment with tone and emphasis until you are satisfied with the way the induction sounds.

2. Choose a location free of any sounds that may be picked up on the tape, such as clocks, television, telephone, or doorbell. You will also need to alert your family or roommates. Make sure they understand that they are not to interrupt you or make any other sounds that can be heard on tape.

3. Put on comfortable clothing and get into a comfortable position. You may want to lie down, sit in a rocking chair, or sit at your desk with your feet up. Whatever your preferred position, make sure it is one that will be comfortable throughout the entire recording session. If you are shifting around or feeling physically uncomfortable, this discomfort will be reflected in the tone and quality of your voice.

Six Sleep Induction Steps

Step 1. Beginning the induction.
The induction begins by focusing your attention on your breathing and inner sensations. As you focus inward, your awareness of external surroundings will decrease. By breathing deeply, you become aware of your internal sensations. You introduce your body to relaxation. Your pulse slows, your breathing slows, you begin to withdraw, and you can direct your attention to the suggestions that are given to you.

Step 2. Systematic relaxation of the body.
As the induction directs you to concentrate on relaxing every muscle in your body, your mind will also become more relaxed. You will experience an increased awareness of internal functions and an increased receptivity of the senses.

Step 3. Creating imagery of deeper relaxation.
The induction's image of drifting down deeper and deeper helps you to enter a deeper trance. Tension in your shoulders is re-

leased by an image of weight being lifted from your shoulders. Any difference in your bodily sensations will support the suggestion that a change is taking place. It does not matter whether the direction specified in the induction is upward or downward, so long as the image of rising or descending makes it possible for you to experience a change in your physical feelings.

Step 4. Deepening the trance.

To help you deepen your trance, or "go down," count backward from ten to one. In order to return to full consciousness, or "come up," count forward from one to ten. The induction uses the image of a staircase with ten steps, but you can substitute any image you like in order to enhance the feeling of going down. The image of an elevator descending ten floors is a popular alternative.

At this stage your limbs may become limp. Your attention will have narrowed, and suggestibility will heighten. The surrounding environment will be closed out.

Step 5. The special place.

The special place you choose to imagine will be one that is unique to you and your experience. It can be a place you have actually visited or one that you imagine. The place does not have to be real, or even possible. You can be sitting on a big blue pillow floating on the surface of a quiet sea. You can be stretched out in a hammock suspended in space. You can be in a cave of clouds. Wherever it is, your special place needs to be one in which you can experience positive feelings and feel safe. It is in this special place that you will have an increased receptivity to further suggestions. That is, once a peaceful feeling is established, you will respond to imagery that reinforces and supports posthypnotic suggestions. Make sure, as you visualize your special place that you try to include sights, sounds, and physical sensations (temperature, texture) in the image.

Step 6. Suggesting sleep.

Now you begin to put away your worries and negative thoughts. You suggest that you are drifting into a sound and restful sleep. You may also add here your own customized suggestion to encourage a deep, refreshing sleep.

Customize Your Induction for Sleep

The following is a list of specific sleep instructions that can be inserted into the induction after you feel yourself settled, centered, and receptive. Or, you can write your own.

I will stay asleep all night.
I won't wake up until it's time.
I will waken refreshed and alert.
Falling asleep is my signal that I am out of a trance and going into deep sleep.
I will get up in the night to use the bathroom if needed, but I will fall asleep again easily.
All thoughts of daytime anxieties are unnecessary; I am allowing them to pass through my conscious awareness and disappear.
I will dream as usual. (Hypnosis will not affect my dreams.)
I will gradually become drowsier and drowsier. In just a few minutes I will be able to fall asleep, and sleep peacefully all night.
I can turn off anger and guilt because I am the one who turns it *on.* I will relax my body and breathe deeply.
Write your own: _____

Hypnotic Induction for Insomnia

The following is adapted from *Hypnosis for Change* by Josie Hadley and Carol Staudacher, 2d ed., New Harbinger Publications, 1989.

Take a nice deep breath, close your eyes, and begin to relax. Just think about relaxing every muscle in your body from the top of your head to the tips of your toes. Just begin to relax. And begin to notice how very comfortable your body is beginning to feel. You are supported, so you can just let go and relax. Inhale and exhale. Notice your breathing; notice the rhythm of your breathing and relax your breathing for a moment.

Be aware of normal sounds around you. These sounds are unimportant, discard them, whatever you hear from now on will only help to relax you. And as you exhale, release any tension, any stress from any part of your body, mind, and thought; just let that stress go. Just feel any stressful thoughts rushing through your mind, feel them begin to wind down, wind down, wind down, and relax.

And begin with letting all the muscles in your face relax, especially your jaw; let your teeth part just a little bit and relax this area. This is a place where tension and stress gather, so be sure to relax your jaw and feel that relaxation go into your temples. Relax the muscles in your temples and as you think about relaxing these muscles they will relax. Feel them relax and as you relax you'll be able to just drift and float into a deeper and deeper level of total relaxation. You will continue to relax, and now let all of the muscles in your forehead relax. Feel those muscles become smooth, smooth, and relaxed, and rest your eyes. Just imagine your eyelids feeling so comfortable, so heavy, so heavy, so relaxed.

And now let all of the muscles in the back of your neck and shoulders relax, feel a heavy, heavy weight being lifted off your shoulders, and you feel relieved, lighter, and more relaxed. And all of the muscles in the back of your neck and shoulders relax, and feel that soothing relaxation go down your back, down, down, down, to the lower part of your back, and feel those muscles let go and with every breath you inhale just feel your body drifting, floating, down deeper, down deeper, down deeper into total relaxation.

Let your muscles go, relaxing more and more. Let all the muscles in your shoulders, running down your arms to your fingertips, relax. And let your arms feel so heavy, so heavy, so heavy, so comfortable, so relaxed. You may have tingling in your fingertips. That's perfectly fine. You may have warmth in the palms of your hands, and that's fine. And you may feel that you can barely lift your arms, they are so relaxed, they are so heavy, so heavy, so relaxed. And now you inhale once again and relax your chest muscles. And now as you exhale, feel your stomach muscles relax. As you exhale, relax all the muscles in your stomach, let them go, and all the muscles in your legs, feel them relax, and all of the muscles in your legs, so completely relaxed right to the tips of your toes.

Notice how very comfortable your body feels, just drifting and floating, deeper, deeper, deeper, relaxed. And as you are relaxing deeper and deeper, imagine a beautiful staircase. There are ten steps, and the steps lead you to a special and peaceful and beautiful place. In a moment you can begin to imagine taking a safe and gentle and easy step down, down, down on the staircase, leading you to a very peaceful, a very special place for you. You can imagine it to be any place you choose, perhaps you would enjoy a beach or ocean with clean, fresh air, or the mountains with a stream; any place is perfectly fine.

In a moment I'm going to count backward from ten to one and you can imagine taking the steps down and as you take each step, feel your body relax, more and more, feel it just drift down, down each step, and relax even deeper,

ten, relax even deeper, nine . . . eight . . . seven . . . six . . .
five . . . four . . . three . . . two . . . one . . . deeper, deeper,
deeper, relaxed. And now imagine a peaceful and special
place. You can imagine this special place and perhaps you
can even feel it. You are in (insert your special place). You
are alone and there is no one to disturb you. This is the
most peaceful place in the world for you. Imagine yourself
there and feel that sense of peace flow through you and
a sense of well-being and enjoy these positive feelings and
keep them with you. Allow these positive feelings to grow
stronger and stronger, feeling at peace with that sense of
well-being. And now just linger in your special place. There
is no place to go, nothing to do. Just rest and let yourself
drift and float, drift and float into a sound and restful
sleep. Just let yourself drift deeper and deeper into sleep.

And now become aware of how comfortable you feel,
so relaxed, your head and shoulders are in just the right
position, your back is supported, and you are becoming
less and less aware of all the normal sounds of your surroundings, and as you drift deeper and deeper you may experience a negative thought or worry trying to surface in
your mind, trying to disrupt your slumber, trying to disrupt your rest. Simply take that thought, sweep it up as you
would sweep up crumbs from the floor and place that
thought or worry into a box. The box has a nice tight lid.
Put the lid on the box and place the box on the top shelf of
your closet. You can go back to that box at another time, a
time that is more appropriate, a time that will not interfere
with your sleep. So as these unwanted thoughts appear,
sweep them up and place them in the box, put a lid on
the box and place it on the top shelf of your closet and let
them go. Let them go and continue to drift deeper and
deeper into sleep.

Shift your thoughts back to your positive thoughts and positive statements. Just let these thoughts flow through your mind, thoughts such as "I am a worthwhile person." (Pause.) "I have accomplished many good things." (Pause.) "I have reached positive goals." (Pause.) Just let your own positive ideas flow through your mind. Let them flow and drift, becoming stronger and stronger as you drift, becoming stronger and stronger as you drift deeper and deeper into sleep. You may begin to see them slowly fade, slowly fade as you become even more relaxed, more sleepy, more drowsy, more relaxed. Just imagine yourself in your peaceful and special place, smiling, feeling so good, so comfortable, so relaxed. (Pause.) And from your special place you can easily drift into a sound and restful sleep, a sound and restful sleep, undisturbed in a sound and restful sleep. You sleep throughout the night in a sound and restful sleep.

If you should awaken simply imagine your special place once again, and drift easily back into a sound and restful sleep, a sound and restful sleep. Your breathing becomes so relaxed, your thoughts wind down, wind down, wind down, and relax. You drift and float into a sound and restful sleep, undisturbed throughout the night. You will awaken at your designated time feeling rested and refreshed.

Now there's nothing to do, nothing to think about, nothing to do but enjoy your special place, your special place that is so peaceful for you, so relaxing. Just imagine how it feels to relax in your special place. You may become aware of how clean and fresh your special place smells, or you may become aware of the different sounds of your special place, such as birds singing in the background, or water cascading over rocks in a stream. Or you may become aware of how warm the sun feels as you lounge in a hammock, or how cool the breeze feels from the ocean air. Or you may experience something else that is unique and wonderful in your special place. Just experience it, drift and float, all thoughts just fading, drifting into a sound and restful sleep. Just drift into a comfortable, cozy, restful sleep, your body feeling heavy and relaxed as you sink into your bed, so relaxed, just drifting into sleep (pause), sleep (pause), sleep (Pause. Softly repeat sleep three more times), sleep . . . sleep . . . sleep . . .

Posthypnotic Suggestions

A cornerstone of the self-hypnotic technique is to introduce posthypnotic suggestions into your trance statements. These suggestions, which are given during the induction and carried out at some other time in the day, serve as cues to reinforce your sleep goals. For example, you may give yourself the suggestion that whenever you see a clock, you are reminded of your growing sense of mastery and control over your insomnia. Posthypnotic cues are most effective if they're incorporated into your daily pre-bed rituals. Dr. Brian Alman, in his book *Self-Hypnosis: A Complete Manual for Health and Self-Change,* suggests that you give yourself these posthypnotic suggestions while in a trance:

"I may notice that when I brush my teeth in the evening, just before bed, as I clean my teeth I can also clean my mind of worry, tension, and anxiety."

"As I take off my robe and hang it on the hook, I may also imagine that on my robe are pinned all of my problems, troubles, and worries from the day. I can see them now, like index cards or signs upon which are written all the worries that might keep me from sleeping. They're too small to read, but I feel that as I lift off my robe the weight of these worries and anxieties are lifted off me also. The robe and these worries are in the closet, and I can put them on tomorrow if I wish. But tonight I can sleep without them."

Meditation and Self-Hypnosis for Napping

For those of you with chronic insomnia, you may want to consider avoiding naps altogether. However, a low point in the body's natural rhythms generally occurs between 2 P.M. and 5 P.M., encouraging that napping feeling each day. Some people, if they have the luxury, are greatly refreshed by a respite from the day's events at this time. Others feel that they are unable to relax enough to take a nap. If you know that you would feel refreshed by a nap, but worry that it might last too long or disrupt your nighttime sleep, you can use self-hypnosis and meditation as tools to facilitate and regulate these breaks. The relaxed state can even serve as a satisfying replacement for napping. Some people find that napping can sometimes take the pressure off their minds about sleeping at night as well, and therefore are more able to sleep when it's time to go to bed.

The idea is to suggest to yourself that you will keep your "nap" brief (ten to twenty minutes). You won't actually fall into sleep, but use the induction techniques just before sleep to relax yourself. You'll find that using meditation and self-hypnosis in this way can be invigorating, whereas falling into a deep sleep can leave you groggy and fatigued for the rest of the day.

If you are a student studying for exams and feel forced to sleep in shifts, you can try using these meditative/self-hypnotic breaks to energize yourself and supplement your sleep. Or if you're a shift worker and find that you have to grab sleep when you can, you may want to try to adapt one of these inductions to help you relax more quickly and efficiently. Choose one of the inductions in this chapter to enter the trance, and insert the following suggestion while in the trance:

> "Now that I am relaxed and comfortable, I know that I can slip easily into sleep. However, I choose instead to remain in this refreshing state, peaceful and aware. As I gradually leave this state and reenter wakefulness, I will feel refreshed, alert, and ready for the rest of the day.
>
> "I can return to a refreshed and alert state by counting from one to five. As I get closer to five my eyes will open. . . . I will feel more refreshed and more alert. One . . . two . . . three . . . four . . . five. . . . I am awake, alert, and feeling good."

Visualization

Your imagination can be a powerful ally and friend in your quest for inner calm. Tribal people throughout the world have used images (of spirits, things natural and unnatural) to invoke pleasure, as well as fear. We literal Americans are skeptics when it comes to believing in the power of things unseen. But athletes, for example, welcome the power of visualization. You will see them mentally rehearsing the "game" or their sport before they actually go on. This use of imagery helps calm them and focuses them to eliminate de-energizing distractions and to do their best.

Visualization is a natural part of meditation and self-hypnosis. Mental pictures you create spontaneously or deliberately will enhance your calm and focused state of mind. These pictures can be literal, such as picturing an escalator going down to help you relax and deepen your trance or meditative state. Or these pictures can be symbolic of overall pleasant feelings, such as the feeling you get when you see, hear, and smell ocean waves crashing upon the beach.

Once you appreciate the power of visualizing images, you are free to experiment with as many images as possible. Just make sure that they are positive, pleasurable images that make you feel good. You might check to see if they make you feel "too good," as in excited, where you want to pop up and finish writing that piece of music, choreographing the dance, painting the picture. Or, you may find in your stillness that a solution to a problem comes to you. This kind of creativity or energy could be a good thing— go with it! If practical, write down the solution, then return to your meditative state. Chances are your body will feel an accomplishment that helps to relax you even more.

If negative, self-defeating images pop into your mind, don't berate yourself, squeezing your eyes tight and trying to force them out of your head. Instead, use the following imagery to "allow" them to pass out of your consciousness:

See the negative words or images go floating past you one by one, each one on a log bobbing slowly on a stream. The stream flows away from you and the logs bob out of sight. See each negative word or image pasted on a balloon. Feel a gentle breeze on your face. See the balloons blow back and forth in the air, finally being carried up and off into the sky.

If you try to force unpleasant thoughts away and they insist on returning, you may find yourself getting more frustrated and aroused by the minute. This only makes it harder for you to relax. Simply repeat the above techniques over and over, without condemning yourself for having the thoughts in the first place. You'll find that your negative thoughts will slowly fade, leaving a smooth running stream or a calm sky in their place to symbolize your blank mind at rest.

Patrick Fanning, author of *Visualization for Change,* an excellent step-by-step guide to using your powers of imagination for self-improvement, includes a section on obsessive ruminations in his insomnia chapter. If you find yourself ruminating obsessively, he suggests trying to keep your mind busy with an elaborate but pleasant visualization. Imagine conducting an orchestra in your favorite piece of music, watching your favorite sports team play a game, choreographing a ballet or jazz dance, building a fancy piece of furniture, sewing a coat—any long, positive, engaging process that will distract you from your other train of thought. I find this to be particularly helpful, as one who obsesses frequently, and so I build my next house in my visualization. I go over each room, detail by detail. If I find I have reached the end of the imagery (I'm out the back door gazing up at my mansion and am still not asleep), then I go back and start over again, this time picking out colors for each room. And, as my husband would say, shoes to match the décor.

Remember not to criticize your choice of images. Let them flow freely, and with practice you'll find that they become richer and more vivid. Incorporate into your trance an image of yourself sleeping successfully throughout the night, awakening alert and refreshed in the morning. See yourself as confident and in control of your situation. See yourself following the suggestions in this book with dedicated intention. See yourself as successful, and you will be.

5

Reconditioning Insomnia

Your body responds best to a regular, daily routine. But in modern society there are many temptations to skip routine. It used to be that people went to sleep when it got dark; the regular cycles of night and day routinized their sleep schedules. Now there is good quality lighting available for reading, working, or using the computer. Television offers an endless supply of visual, often mindless distraction. Social changes have had as much impact as technological changes. For instance, interest, education, and economic necessity have merged to encourage many women to work full-time outside of the home. Late nights may be the only hours available to catch up on household matters or to spend concentrated time with family members. Regardless of gender, being "perfect" is still a goal in success-oriented America. For too many people, that means sacrificing sleep in an effort to "get there."

Aside from cutting into sleep hours, all this late-night activity may wake you up rather than calm you down enough to go to sleep. In your efforts to be a perfect person, do you find yourself memorizing things you have to do the next day while lying in bed? This is a common example of inappropriately using your bed as an "activity center," or a place where wakeful things are going on that are incompatible with sleepiness. Dr. Hauri calls this *conditioned insomnia*, where a

71

kind of "unconscious learning" sets in. You have learned to associate your bed and bedtime with wakefulness. Examples of other incompatible nighttime behaviors in the bed or the bedroom are:

arguing
lively discussion
eating
reading exciting books
exercising
cleaning
worrying
talking on the phone
watching TV

Your pre-bed ritual can contain very powerful associations that cue sleepiness. Brushing your teeth, setting the clock, arranging the covers: all can signal sleep time. However, if you associate your bed with stimulating activities such as eating, arguing, or watching TV—sexual activity excepted—you may actually have trained yourself to be wakeful rather than sleepy.

The last one, watching TV, is debatable, because some people are lulled to sleep throughout the night by the drone of TV, especially if the volume is kept low.

Athletes condition their bodies through regular training. They work to establish positive habits toward a greater goal. But negative patterns or habits can be learned, too. Insomnia can be "conditioned" through associations you develop either consciously or unconsciously. Although you may enjoy the change of pace of a spontaneous late-night movie or intimate discussion, be aware that if you repeatedly encourage poor habits, you may unwittingly invite insomnia. Instead, you can train your body, much as an athlete does, to respond to certain cues and adopt specific habits to help you perform better. This chapter helps you look at destructive associations you may make and suggests ways for you to decondition those associations.

For example, one business executive finds herself running through the next day's activities each night before she forces her eyes shut. She begins to dread her bed because she associates it with a time for mental rehearsal. Her planning and worrying only remind her of unaccomplished tasks and thus of her imperfections. Another scenario: a freelance artist uses the quiet night to write. She takes restful but lengthy naps to compensate for lost sleep. After a time, she finds that the slant of the late afternoon sun "cues" her nap time. When she's ready to return to a steady job, it's exceedingly difficult to reprogram her body to do without the nap. In both examples certain stimuli (anxious thoughts, naps in the sun) cue certain behaviors (difficulty adapting to "normal" sleep patterns). As time passes, those behaviors become increasingly ingrained and destructive.

In 1972 a psychologist named Dr. Richard Bootzin pioneered work in stimulus control for insomnia. The above issues are just the ones he considered: what cues are established prior to sleepiness and surrounding the sleep area. Dr. Bootzin determined that a primary goal for the insomnia sufferer is to associate the bed *solely* with sleep, nothing else. The idea makes sense when you consider the many insomniacs who dread their bed because they see it as a place to toss, turn, and worry—and who then find that their sleep is better when they travel, or even move into a different room. In a new setting, their typical nonsleep cues are absent, and they sleep peacefully.

The cornerstone of stimulus control treatment for insomnia is working to create a "new" setting of your own bed. You want it to be associated solely and clearly with restful sleep. This means methodically eliminating all negative associations. The following guidelines based on Dr. Bootzin's recommendations will help you achieve this goal.

1. Go to bed *only* when you feel sleepy. If you go to bed too early and then toss and turn, you will experience the feelings of frustration that you want to avoid.
2. Do not use your bed as an activity center. Sexual activity is the only exception. For a list of examples of inappropriate activities, see the beginning of this chapter.
3. If you do not fall asleep in about ten to twenty minutes, get out of bed and go into another room. Do a nonarousing activity until you feel sleepy. Only when you feel drowsy should you go back to bed.
4. If *again* you do not fall asleep in about ten to twenty minutes, get up; repeat your nonarousing activity or try another one. Do not return to bed until you feel sleepy.
5. Repeat as often as necessary until you feel yourself falling easily asleep. Your goal is to associate your bed with falling asleep with ease.
6. Get up the same time each morning, regardless of how little you slept. This is a very important step. A consistent uptime will help your body begin to develop a regular sleep rhythm. Resist the temptation to break conditioning by sleeping late on weekend mornings.
7. Do not nap. Your goal is to establish consistent sleep cues at regular times; napping can disrupt your sleep cues.
8. If all else fails, try sleeping in a different room or moving your bed to a different location in your room.

Common Obstacles to This Approach

At first it will feel uncomfortable to jump in and out of bed throughout the night. You may resist leaving a warm bed, especially on cold winter nights. Or you may resent the loneliness of a dark, quiet house. You may even feel particularly fatigued and sluggish for the first few days of trying this approach. Some people complain that they feel even *worse* than usual at the start of this strategy.

These reactions are common and understandable. But be assured that this process has been used successfully for many patients over many years and has helped chronic insomniacs reshape attitudes toward their beds and sleep. Dr. Bootzin found that 57 percent of the patients in one study who learned this stimulus control training eventually averaged less than twenty-five minutes a night to fall asleep. This is an impressive success rate, especially when compared to a 29 percent "success" for those who used Progressive Muscle Relaxation (PMR), 27 percent for those who relied on self-relaxation techniques, and 22 percent for the control subjects who received no treatment. Although it is wise for you not to expect immediate improvement, some people have found that they are able to sleep better within a week of carefully following stimulus control techniques. With consistent effort you will find that the sleep you gain in the long run will more than compensate for the sleep you lose those first few nights.

After working with Dr. Bootzin's stimulus control program for some time, another researcher developed a list of suggestions that helped her patients succeed in the program. Dr. Patricia Lacks of St. Louis, Missouri, led patients through the stimulus control treatment plan over a four-week period, within the context of a support group. The list below includes those strategies that the group found to be most helpful.

Suggestions for Success

1. While up at night, avoid any activities that might promote alertness. Examples might be finishing a novel or movie to see how it ends or doing work brought home from the office. Choose something that can be easily discontinued after two

minutes, fifteen minutes, or two hours—whenever you feel sleepy. For ideas on mundane things to do, see chapter 15.

2. Avoid unconsciously "punishing" yourself for not sleeping by forcing yourself to do an unpleasant activity. It will be much harder to get out of the bed if you think you have to face the laundry or the unbalanced checkbook.

3. Make it easier on yourself to get out of bed by leaving a cozy bathrobe and flashlight nearby. This way you can slip out without disturbing your partner. The house will also seem less dark, cold, and unfriendly.

4. Avoid eating. If you must snack, eat a light food containing carbohydrates, calcium, soy, or dairy products. Do *not* indulge in sugar, alcohol, caffeine, or any other stimulating foods.

5. Don't worry about following the ten-minute rule to the precise second. Estimate the ten-minute period. The point is, if you find yourself lying in bed fully awake after a reasonable amount of time, get up. But if you estimate that it's been twenty minutes and you feel yourself dropping off to sleep, stay there. Avoid clock watching.

6. Tell yourself to get up when the alarm clock rings, no matter how restless your night has been. This is an important step. Remember, you want to reregulate your internal associations and settle your body into a steady rhythm.

7. Record your progress with reconditioning your insomnia in your sleep diary. Keeping a careful record of your sleep progress and behavior will help you gain perspective on your problem. You may spot patterns or connections you had not noticed before. Also, you'll feel a sense of mastery and hope as you see yourself making progress. For a sample diary, see the end of chapter 2, "Sleep Hygiene."

You will need to be diligent in following all of the above guidelines in order to break the vicious cycle of your negative associations. But pace yourself; do not expect miracles overnight. Allow yourself time to gradually comprehend and adopt the principles you find in this chapter. If you find that this technique does not work for you, don't panic. You may be one of those who prefers to adopt one of the other techniques found in this book, such as meditation, or gradual muscle relaxation. In any case, making use of the sleep diary will help coordinate your plan of action. Share it with a trusted friend or a health-care professional. Ask for support and encouragement. Success can be sweeter when shared with another who supports your accomplishments.

6

Managing Obsessions

This chapter is about your thought processes and how they affect your ability to cope with insomnia. Before you give in to the temptation to skip over this chapter and move on to the next one (saying this "doesn't apply to me"), keep an open mind and read on. Don't dismiss your mind's ability to affect your body, and blame everything on external stress or a physical ailment. Your mind is a powerful tool that can work to keep you awake all night, or that can be harnessed to help you cope more effectively and sleep.

A common lament heard by poor sleepers is "I can't sleep!" Obviously they are lamenting the immediate inability to fall asleep, but there is a hidden message in the phrase "I can't sleep!" That message is one of hopelessness, despair, inability to *ever* make anything right. In other words, "I can't make it right. I can't sleep!" has a helpless certainty to it that defies flexibility and openness to challenge. Out of frustration and anxiety, the utterer of this phrase not only can't sleep but *won't* sleep.

Insomniacs have a fine ability to obsess. They take this tendency to bed, and lie there ruminating about their own and others' shortcomings. For example, rather than move away from anger to problem solving, insomniacs will replay the situation that caused them such anger, over and over. Or, they will end-lessly count the ways they, or others, are imperfect.

An underlying issue of any illness or physical disorder is the thought process you bring to the situation. With physical pain, how you think about your pain determines your ability to cope with it. If chronic insomniacs think in a negative way about ever sleeping better, their prophecies will become self-fulfilling. If you find yourself thinking, "I'll never get better," "This shouldn't have happened to me," "I'm so embarrassed that I have this prob-lem; I must be less of a person," then you are doing yourself a dis-service. You are predetermining that you will *never* improve.

Obsessional Characteristics of Insomniacs

Studies show that insomniacs tend to be anxious, stressed, and prone to perfectionistic tendencies. Failure is difficult for them to accept, in their own or in others' behavior. Consequently, when others are sleeping peacefully, they lie in bed rerunning the day's events, wishing they had said or done something else, trying to avert future catastrophes, and so on.

Insomniacs tend to be physically tense people—they tighten muscles automatically in response to excitement. In turn, they are prone to illness and other physical complaints. The NSF re-ports that as scientists learn more about the function of sleep, a growing body of research is making the connection between in-adequate sleep and the increased risk of a number of health con-ditions, such as type 2 diabetes and hypertension. For example, a study published by the University of Chicago in 1999 showed that a sleep debt of three to four hours a night over the course of a week affected the health of young, healthy males. Their bodies were less able to process carbohydrates, manage stress, and main-tain a proper balance of hormones.

Another study published in 2000 in the *Journal of the American Medical Association* found that lack of sleep impacted the production of a certain growth hormone, linking that to a propensity for obesity later in the subjects' lives.

Insomniacs also tend toward rigidity and inflexibility. When things do not happen as they "should," or in precise order, insomniacs tense up and dwell on the problem obsessively. They obsess about mistakes, problems, plans, and future uncertainties. If you suspect that you fall into any of these categories, you are probably familiar with the following typical pattern: as you experience difficulty falling asleep, you begin to be concerned about losing sleep. You say to yourself things like: "Oh, no . . . not again." Or, "Here I go again," "How can I keep doing this?" or, "I won't be alert for the meeting tomorrow."

These initial thoughts set up a chain reaction. You tense up in response to these negative thoughts, which then makes it harder to relax enough to go to sleep. You may say to yourself, "I must go to sleep," or, "I should try harder," which only sets you up for feelings of failure when you don't perform. You may notice that you can fall asleep much more easily when you're not trying, such as when you're watching TV. High expectations of self are typical of the insomniac. You expect perfection of yourself in every aspect, which leaves no room for the weakness of not being able to sleep on command.

To sum it all up, see if you can spot yourself in the following eight general characteristics of insomniacs:

1. You have a history of general physical arousal. Your body becomes tensed and you typically react with stress to excitement, both negative and positive.
2. You have a specific tendency toward high muscle tension under stress. You clench your teeth and tighten muscles,

which may bring on tension headaches, back pain, fatigue, and general muscular aches.

3. You have a fear of failure. The notion of failing at anything is totally unacceptable to you.

4. You suffer from perfectionistic tendencies. You cannot allow yourself to be less than perfect, which means you "fail" when you don't sleep well.

5. You are angry. You carry anger with you to the bedroom. The anger affects not only your sleep, but your work and home relationships.

6. You tend to turn everything into a catastrophe. Your perfectionistic standards and fear of failing combine to put you constantly on the defensive. You can expect the worst to come true of most things and people around you, and you worry about what you'll do when it does.

7. You have a fear of letting go. This means that you cannot let down your guard, for fear that events and people will escape your control. You must remain ever vigilant.

8. You obsess. Because of your tendencies toward all of the above, you dwell on problems and issues, trying to solve them by incessant worrying.

Steps You Can Take to Counteract Negative, Obsessional Thinking

Step 1: Awareness

Even if negative, obsessional thinking impedes your progress toward better sleep, you can take steps to harness that thinking and change it into something that works for you, rather than against you. Your first step is to become aware of your own patterns of obsessional thinking. For one full week, notice obsessional thoughts creeping into your mind, day or night, and jot them down. How many are there? What are they about? Are they linked to a particular situation, or do they spontaneously occur? What does your body physically do as you think these thoughts? (e.g., do you clench your fists, your jaw?) As you drop off to sleep or wake up in the middle of the night, have paper and pencil by your bedside to help you keep track of all these thoughts. You might also have a flashlight or book light handy so as not to disturb your bedmate. You may find it helpful to use the sleep diary form in chapter 2. Or, buy a small notebook to use exclusively to chart your sleep progress.

You can use the following shorthand to label each brand of thinking:

FAIL—fear of failing
PERF—tendency toward perfectionism
ANGER—general anger
CATA—expecting the worst, "the what ifs?"
GO—inability to let things go
OBSESS—constant worrying

After one full week, review your notes. Which brand of obsessional thinking do you do the most? Are there any patterns in your thinking?

You may find that you have many other types of thoughts that do not fit neatly into the categories provided here. Simply write them down in your own words and become familiar with them. The purpose is to provide yourself a framework within which to work, so that the prospect of controlling negative thinking does not seem overwhelming.

Step 2: Stop Your Thoughts
After you feel more fully aware of your style of obsessional thinking, you can begin to counteract each thought. Negative thinking arrives with such spontaneity and fury that you will need to arm

yourself with as much counterammunition as possible. The ammunition will take the form of positive thoughts delivered with equal force and significance.

Steps to Thought Stopping

As soon as you notice that you are obsessing negatively, choose a way to abruptly halt the unproductive flow of thinking. The following statements are designed to replace each negative thought. Read them over thoroughly. You may not agree with them at first. This is natural and perfectly acceptable. However, in order for you not to continually lose sleep because you obsess, you will need to find an agreeable replacement, a statement in which you can believe. The counteracting statements that follow are just examples. You may find that you get best results from developing your own healthy rejoinders to the negative thoughts. Use the blank lines under the counteracting statements to write your own rejoinders.

Don't forget to check the physical sensations that accompany your negative thoughts. For example, do you grit your teeth, clench your fists, hold your breath? These reactions may even be unconscious, so pay attention to your body, and allow yourself to physically relax as you practice your counteracting statements.

Examples of Counteracting Statements

1. When you feel yourself tensing up, say to yourself:
   "I can relax."
   "My muscles are becoming limp."
   "I am calmer."
   "Breathe deeply."
   My suggestions: _____
   Follow the directions in chapter 3, "Relaxation for Sleep"
   for more instructions on relaxation strategies.

2. When you find yourself obsessing about failure, think about examples of successes in advance. When obsessing on failures at night, shift focus to an example of success and say to yourself:

"Sometimes I succeed, sometimes I don't. Time to relax and sleep."

"I am not a failure."

"I have succeeded in life before."

"Just because I can't sleep tonight doesn't mean I'm a failure."

"I will not suffer tomorrow if I lose sleep tonight."

My suggestions: _____

3. When you become aware of your perfectionist mind-set, think of phrases like:

"It's okay to be less than perfect."

"No one says I have to be perfect."

"There is no such thing as a perfect person, and if there were, that person would be very boring."

"Enough kicking myself for one night. Things will look different in the morning."

My suggestions: _____

4. When you notice yourself feeling angry:

"I will leave my anger outside of the bedroom."

"All these things making me angry will be waiting for me tomorrow. I can deal with them then."

"Let go of angry thoughts. Time to relax."

My suggestions: _____

5. When you notice that you are expecting the worst about some upcoming event or your life in general, think of statements like:

"It's impossible that everything will work out for the worst."

"It's possible things will work out for the best"

"Things will be the same whether I worry or not."

"Other people have their own issues—they are not out to get me."

"Everything seems worse in the middle of the night."

My suggestions: _____

6. When you realize that you are trying too much to control some situation or set of circumstances, these statements can help you loosen your grip on things:

"I am learning not to have to control everything."

"Stay flexible. I've done what I can: the rest is up to fate."

"Go with the flow."

"Don't sweat the small stuff, and it's all small stuff!"

My suggestions: _____

7. When you notice you are obsessively rerunning statements or events, you can say to yourself:

"I will counteract each negative thought with a peaceful, soothing thought."

"I will not let these thoughts drive me crazy."

"I will dismiss them one by one, and replace them with thoughts that will help me feel sleepy."

"I see my negative thoughts floating like autumn leaves on the surface of a stream, drifting around the bend and out of sight."

My suggestions: _____

Replacing your negative thinking takes time, patience, practice, and commitment. Don't give up if you don't notice immediate improvement in sleep onset and quality. You've spent a lifetime collecting your own unique brand of negative thought; allow yourself time to unravel it and develop better habits.

You will find that using visualization to augment your thinking can add power to your thoughts. Visualize yourself as a powerful, confident, and relaxed person. See yourself speaking assertively. Imagine yourself cool under pressure. Re-create feelings of pleasure at your success at staying cool, assertive, and confident. Some people experience great success choosing positive scenes or objects, ones that evoke feelings of peace, calm, and nurturing support. See chapter 4 for more information on visualization.

Everything Seems Worse at Night

This technique of replacing negative thoughts can work at any time, day or night, whenever you notice yourself becoming anxious and full of worries. All you have to do is practice enough, and it will become second nature to react positively rather than negatively. A particularly vulnerable time of the night is in the predawn hours—3 A.M. to 5 A.M.—when it's easy to feel overtaken by anxious thoughts. If you awaken frequently during these hours and have difficulty getting back to sleep, prepare yourself before you go to bed each night to administer positive phrases to yourself as soon as necessary.

7

Circadian Rhythms and Sleep

The word "circadian" comes from *circa,* a derivative of the Latin word *circum* (around, about) and *dies* (also Latin, for day), and means "about one day." In the 1940s and '50s, researchers strove to determine human sleeping and waking cycles. These cycles came to be known as circadian cycles or rhythms. Dr. Nathaniel Kleitman, often called the father of modern sleep research, once stated that sleep is "part of a perpetual cycle and the most powerful organizer of our lives." When you fall out of sync with your body's natural, daily cycle, you and your day are disrupted.

Your daily rhythms are synchronized with your body's internal and external cues. The primary internal cue is your inner "body clock," which regulates certain physiological functions such as body temperature and hormone levels. A body clock is one way to picture the control of the circadian rhythm. Examples of other bodily functions that reflect cyclic changes are heart rate, blood pressure, endocrine secretions, metabolism, breathing, and associated mood swings.

External cues include the amount of sunlight available and the "social clock," or daily activities such as mealtimes. If time is distorted, as when you travel across time zones or are forced to lose sleep, your body's rhythm falls out of sync with its environment.

The results can be very unsettling: difficulty falling asleep, restless and disturbed sleep, and fatigue and disorientation the following day.

Common causes of circadian rhythm disruption are:

1. Insomnia due to self-imposed sleep-wake schedule disruption. An example might be a student cramming for exams and limiting sleep to naps or to hourly increments.
2. Insomnia related to shift work or night work.
3. Rapid time-zone change syndrome, also known as "jet lag," and sometimes referred to as "transmeridian travel sleep disorder."

Your Internal Time Clock

Human circadian rhythms in individuals can vary from twenty-four to twenty-eight hours, with a general tendency toward twenty-four to twenty-five hour cycles. During this cycle your body temperature rises and falls in a predictable cycle, which in turn affects when you feel sleepy and when you are ready to be awake and alert. Your clock alarm going off each morning cues your body, as well as dawn and dusk. Since the inherent human rhythm can be a little longer than the twenty-four-hour day, some people instinctively gravitate toward going to bed an hour later and getting up an hour later each day. This has an impact on your ability to adapt to work-shift and time-zone changes, as you will see later in this chapter.

Body temperature fluctuations account for dips and peaks in mental and physical alertness. Temperatures generally are lowest during the latter half of sleep, about 3 A.M. to 5 A.M., when most people need to be the least alert because they are the most deeply asleep. Temperatures rise in the morning, peaking somewhere between midday and the late afternoon, and begin to fall as the

evening hours approach. However, there is a great deal of individual variation in the precise times that people peak during the day.
This may explain why some people are morning people, or "larks,"
and others are night people, or "owls." Larks' temperatures tend to
peak earlier than that of owls. Dr. Kleitman discovered that alertness follows body temperature: you feel most alert and perform
best when body temperature is highest, and least alert when body
temperature is lowest. Of course, external factors can affect these
dips and peaks, such as extreme hot or cold climates, eating and
drinking hot or cold foods, and vigorous exercise. And, no matter
if you're an owl or lark, it seems that everyone is affected by the familiar phenomenon of "postlunch dip." This occurs in most adults
around 2 P.M., and may be a secondary circadian subrhythm having
nothing to do with the amount of lunch you've eaten!

Society expects its members to conform to a twenty-four-hour
cycle, which is usually not a tremendous problem for most people. However, you may notice that on weekends you tend to go
to bed later and get up later, so that by Monday morning you
are slightly out of sync with your usual Monday rising time. This is
the mark of that natural drift toward later bedtimes and uptimes
mentioned earlier. You may simply notice that after a day or two
of working days you are back on your regular schedule, feeling
rested and alert when you awaken.

Some people, however, have serious difficulty adjusting to a
twenty-four-hour cycle. Owls, for example, really don't feel awake
until the late afternoon hours. They reach their peak alertness
sometime in the late evening, when larks are yawning and getting
ready for bed. In contrast, larks feel that their best hours are in
the first half of the day; they usually have a low period in the
afternoon and then are truly ready for sleep between 9 P.M. and
11 P.M. Some theories hold that larks tend to be introverted people, and owls extroverts. (That may just reveal owls' penchant for
late-night parties!)

One freelance artist felt that she produced her best work in the evening hours. She developed the habit of watching late-night TV to relax after an evening's work. However, her spouse's alarm clock went off at the same early hour each morning. To compensate, she woke up late and took restful but lengthy naps in the afternoon. She found it increasingly difficult to go to sleep at a regular hour with her spouse. The artist has a stimulus control problem such as that discussed in chapter 5—her daytime ritual involved a nap and her pre-bed ritual involved late-night TV. Combined with these cues, she also fell into her natural circadian rhythm by allowing herself to go to sleep later and later. In order to get back on a schedule more like her spouse's, she needed to reset her body's clock.

If you choose a family lifestyle and a career that allows you to work at your own rhythm and pace, sleep-wake schedules may not be an issue. But if you suspect that part of your insomnia is due to unsynchronized schedules, you may want to discuss this problem further with a specialist at a sleep lab. Sometimes known as "chronotherapists," these specialists can carefully examine your individual sleep-wake schedule and help you find alternative solutions.

Shift Work Syndrome

Many Americans work night shifts and/or rotating shifts. It is estimated that as many as 15 million Americans have nontraditional work schedules that conflict with their biological clocks, according to a 1991 U.S. Congress, Office of Technology Assessment study. Because of the constantly increasing needs of competitive industry, incentives are given to employees—increased salaries, bonuses, and other advantages—to keep the factories operating at peak around the clock. But little attention is paid to whether workers themselves can operate at peak around the clock. "Most existing work schedules are incompatible with the properties of the human circadian time system," write Drs. Charles Czeisler and James Allan of Harvard Medical School. While working rotating shifts does have advantages, there is a high prevalence of reported sleep complaints in shift workers.

A few of the advantages, besides increased pay, are that shift workers don't have to face the traffic and shopping congestion of normal working hours, and they may have significantly more autonomy on evening or night shifts. But many studies claim greater physical ailments among rotating shift workers. In addition, researchers have found the personal injury rate of rotating shift workers to be two to three times greater than that of permanent day, evening, or night workers. Shift workers also complain of:

irregular eating habits, poor diet
disorientation
fatigue, anxiety
strained family relationships
low morale among coworkers
absenteeism
inability to participate in hobbies/exercise

One expert in this field, Dr. Richard Coleman of Stanford University Medical School, has consulted with many businesses about creative adaptation of shift work to the human circadian rhythm. Shift work is here to stay, he acknowledges. But certain changes can make it less personally disruptive, such as rotating shifts in a clockwise fashion: from days to evenings to nights. This way workers can follow the natural lengthening of their day, based on the average twenty-four-hour cycle. If you went the other way—counterclockwise—you would be cutting back an hour or two each day. Imagine trying to fall asleep earlier, for example by 7 P.M., if your normal bedtime is 11 P.M. You would be fueling sleep onset difficulties.

Dr. Coleman further suggests that shifts last three weeks instead of one. If the rotation period is once a week, shift workers never have a chance to adapt to a new rhythm.

Studies show that when companies adapt shifts to accommodate human circadian rhythms and worker comfort levels, there is a marked improvement in employee health and performance. Some companies have adopted a "rapid rotation" system, in which the shifts are one day, one evening, and one night in a row. In this way the worker does not spend enough time on any one shift to adapt to that shift, and remains primarily on daytime rhythm.

You may choose to be permanently assigned to one shift, such as the night shift. The only problem with a fixed shift is that you still need adjustment time when you revert to everyone else's hours on the weekends. But for the most part you can gradually reset your inner clock to adapt to shift work. In effect you invert the regular sleep-wake schedule so that you are alert at 3 A.M. when others are normally sleepy. Dr. Hauri suggests that in order to reset your internal clock, you choose to shift your cycle to an earlier time frame, forcing yourself to get up when the alarm rings. You cannot force sleepiness, only wakefulness. Rather than trying to go to sleep earlier in order to awaken earlier, go to sleep at your regular time and get less sleep that night. The resulting tiredness will help you fall asleep earlier the next night. Over a period of weeks, you can accomplish a resetting of shifts.

The roughest schedules to adapt to seem to be rotating shifts, in which complete adaptation to the new schedule is never made. The human body seems most comfortable working either straight days or straight nights. If you must work rotating shifts, remember that it may take as many as nine full days to adjust. Also, owls and younger people adapt more readily to shift work.

Jet Lag Syndrome

Since people adapt naturally to going to sleep an hour later and rising an hour later each day, it is usually easier to lengthen days rather than shorten them. This may explain why you feel less disruption in your schedule when you add an hour in the fall, compared to losing an hour in the spring. This may also explain why it's less stressful to travel from east to west. Traveling from New York to California makes your day seem longer; this corresponds to your body's natural tendency. But imagine traveling from New York to Paris and arriving at 9 A.M. With a six-hour time difference, the morning arrival in Europe corresponds to the point at which your body temperature is lowest—and you feel the least responsive and alert. You've also shortened your day, fighting against your internal clock.

Dr. Czeisler reports that before people have adapted to a new time zone, there is an increased risk of accidents, errors, and injuries due to decreased alertness. He cites a study in 1980 by Dr. Timothy Monk, whose research results showed a 10 percent to 11 percent increase in automobile accidents during the week following the introduction of daylight savings time, "which did not occur in certain years when the change was cancelled to conserve energy." Even if you don't travel cross-country, you feel the effects twice a year of a one-hour time difference! The rule of thumb is, for every one-hour time zone you cross, you will need one full day to recover.

These uncomfortable symptoms of jet lag are unforgettable:

fatigue, decreased alertness
loss of appetite
frequent nighttime urination
irresistible sleepiness and/or insomnia
disorientation/sense of confusion
decreased concentration and performance

Frequent flyers, such as airline crews, also report an increase in gastrointestinal disorders and nervousness.

Journeys by ship, bus, or train will *not* have the same effects. Evidently the slower rate of travel allows for adjustment time. You also have to cross time zones to feel the effects of jet lag; traveling from North America to South America, for example, produces no symptoms.

Research shows that those who get out of their hotel rooms and experience greater exposure to light by including outdoor activities adapt more quickly to the new time zone and have less disruption from jet lag. Otherwise, adaptation to the new environment can occur within two days to two weeks.

Suggestions for overcoming jet lag:

Do *not* schedule important meetings immediately upon your arrival; try to arrive a day or two early to recover from jet lag as completely as possible.

You can choose to stay on home time, especially if you are visiting briefly and are able to control activities.

Adopt the social activities of the new time zone upon arrival; go outside, eat meals on local time, stay active, and then turn in earlier. In other words, don't go to your hotel room and go to sleep right away, or you will prolong the adjustment period. Evidence shows that as much exposure to sunlight as possible will aid your adjustment to the new time zone; if you don't feel like walking around, at least sit outside.

Use a short-acting sleeping pill to help you sleep on the first night at your destination (with your doctor's approval).

Anticipate the time zone of your destination by adjusting to its mealtimes, activities, and sleep time wherever possible before your trip. For example, if you are traveling east to west, go to bed and get up an hour later each day for three days before your trip. For west to east travel, move sleep time back an hour earlier each day.

There is not sufficient evidence to prove the claims of a jet lag diet, but some researchers and frequent travelers advocate the following traveler's diet:

Three to four days before departure, alternate meals of high protein, high carbohydrate foods, and fasting-type foods. High protein meals might include cereals, eggs, meat, chicken, or fish. High carbohydrate meals include breads, potatoes, or pasta. Fasting foods include soups, salads, fruits, and juices. The theory is that alternating meals, and the timing of those meals, can help induce shifts to the new time zone. Also, a high protein diet is thought to promote alertness and a high carbohydrate diet to stimulate sleep.

Some people are affected more strongly by jet lag than others. Elderly people, for example, have more difficulty adapting to different time zones. Also, it appears that owls adapt more easily to crossing time zones and experience fewer ill effects in general.

Melatonin

Melatonin is a natural hormone that regulates sleep and wakefulness. Available as an over-the-counter (OTC) product, it has been given as a sleeping pill and proven useful for those people experiencing jet lag. Some researchers have cited tremendous success in treating insomnia, as well, but Dr. Hauri in *No More Sleepless Nights* states that "many experts are still reluctant to recommend melatonin because the sleep-inducing properties have not been well documented and because of its many other actions as a hormone." He further recommends you discuss this with your health-care practitioner, and use it as infrequently and in as low a dosage as possible.

8

Sleep and Dreaming

"Sweet dreams . . . ," your bedmate may whisper to you before drifting off. For many, however, those words are contradictory. If you experience nightmares, dreams are anything but sweet, and may cause sweating, tossing and turning, and a severe dread of sleep. The problem may be as simple as an occasional annoying dream, or it may be a persistent, devastating nocturnal event. It may become a major contribution to your insomnia.

Some people swear they do *not* dream. They rarely if ever recall even a single dream upon awaking. But in fact, humans dream many dreams, averaging about two hours each and every night. Scientists don't know precisely why you dream, much less why you would fail to remember your dreams. Scientists do know, however, that dreams occur to people as elaborate plots that are sometimes meaningful, sometimes nonsensical. Your dream plots may fade to the point that, upon awakening, you are unaware you were even dreaming. In general, it's estimated that dreams occur approximately 80 percent of the time you are in the stage of sleep called rapid eye movement, or REM sleep. REM sleep, so called because the eye rapidly shifts back and forth and up and down during this phase of sleep, occurs about once every ninety minutes in the sleep cycle throughout the night. REM sleep lasts anywhere from three minutes to fifty-five minutes, and there are typically four to six REM periods in a night. That leaves you ample time for dreaming!

REM periods also lengthen as the night wears on, which probably explains why your dreams appear to be so much more vivid and numerous just before you wake up. Dreaming can also occur during the other stages of the sleep cycle, stages one through four, also known as non–REM or NREM sleep. However, these dreams are reported to be more general and vague in nature, with less action and fewer identifiable characters and objects. This may explain why REM dreams are more clearly remembered.

If you dread going to sleep because you fear the return of a disturbing dream, you will benefit from becoming familiar with and desensitized to your dreams. Using the techniques outlined in this chapter, you can learn to welcome the message your dream may be bringing to you. You can learn to escape nightmares in the earliest stages and even turn them into learning experiences. Instead of being experiences to avoid, your dreams can help you unravel daily hassles and deep anxieties that may be contributing to your nightmares.

Why You Dream

Scientists have yet to fully explain the precise reason for dreaming. Some say dreaming is an immense housecleaning effort by the brain, as it chemically sorts out the day's events from past and recent memories—a sort of clearing of the mind's cobwebs. Others downplay the meaning of dreams, saying that they are only a random firing of neurons, or chaotic electrical impulses. The brain seeks to organize these random impulses by affixing images and plots culled from memory or daily experience. In other words, for them, dreams are unlikely harbingers of psychic messages or solutions to problems. Before modern thought and technology afforded a view of actual mental activity, by means of the EEG for example, far more complex philosophies existed to make meaning of dreams.

The ancients often attributed dreams to external sources, although they saw dreams as rich in personal meaning. One of the earliest reports of dream therapy occurred in ancient Greece, when dream healers used "incubation" temples for dreamers to sleep in and work with their dreams. The Greeks believed that dreams brought messages of hope and healing from the gods. Contrast this to other periods in history when dreams were not regarded in a positive light, but were rather considered evil invaders of the body by the devil and bad gods. Sigmund Freud, in the early 1900s, was the first to explore the meaning of dreams from a perspective of unconscious impulses. Freud suggested that the body attempted to "act out" its wishes and desires, often sexual, through dreams. Freud's disciple, Carl Jung, attached a more mystical meaning to dreams, choosing to interpret them as symbols of universal human experience.

Some modern researchers have been drifting toward a behavioral explanation of dreaming. For example, they say that dreaming may be a purely adaptive response, allowing the dreamer to periodically "wake up just a bit" throughout the night to check out the environment. If it is safe, the dreamer can go back to sleep. Richard Coleman writes in *Wide Awake at 3:00 A.M.* that "REM sleep and dreaming may serve as an adaptational process. The amount of REM sleep of newly divorced women has been shown in studies to increase, supporting the theory that dreaming enhances the capacity to cope with emotional problems." Dr. Dement refuses to dismiss dreams as random neuronal events, and concurs with the widespread belief that the dream state reflects the dreamer's real experiences, and that people look to their dreams for profound messages and insight into their lives.

With all the controversy surrounding the origin and purpose of dreaming, two things remain certain:

1. Everyone dreams throughout the night.
2. Dreams provide an opportunity to gain insight into your waking life.

Dream workers have concluded that dream content relates to your core issues, those that you are most concerned about. Joan Mazza writes in *Dreaming Your Real Self* that you always dream about what is most on your mind, and that your core issues will appear in your dreams by way of repeated symbols and recurrent themes. Thinking anxious thoughts and/or engaging in anxiety-provoking activities before bedtime can result in disturbing dreams. Obsessions and desires that haunt you as you lie down to sleep will often find their way into your dreams. For example, laboratory dreams of patients with anorexia nervosa (an eating disorder) contain oral images and preoccupations with food and drink. Ex-smokers will often report vivid dreams of smoking a cigarette for years after they quit.

Several other factors complicate dream content, such as physical condition and substance abuse. Some researchers have found an increase in dream anxiety and hostility during the premenstrual and menstrual phases of a woman's monthly cycle. Others have shown that "REM rebound" occurs with withdrawal from substances such as alcohol and sleeping pills, resulting in frequent and vivid dreams that can seem like nightmares.

It is not surprising, then, that people with vivid and frightening dreams come to dread bedtime. Going to sleep can seem like giving oneself up to the forces of evil. But the dream techniques described in this chapter can help you regain control over your nights. Lucid dreaming, for example, can help you recognize the fact that you are in a dream *while you're still dreaming*—an awareness that alone can ease your fear. Waking fantasy can help you rewrite a troubling ending to a dream. With practice you can find a way out of your nightmares, and even turn them into positive learning experiences. As with other sleep disturbances, such as night terrors and sleepwalking, an effective treatment is really a double cure. It eases the problem itself, and removes the resistance to sleep as well.

Night Terrors, Sleepwalking, and Nightmares

Night terrors, sleepwalking, and nightmares fall into the general category of "parasomnias," or partial arousals throughout the night that disrupt sleep. While night terrors—moments of acute fear or disorientation that are usually forgotten afterward—and sleepwalking most commonly occur in childhood, nightmares are the most common form of parasomnia in adults. Night terrors and sleepwalking have been shrouded in greater mystery than nightmares, although research has gone a long way toward demystifying the phenomena.

Night terrors, sometimes called sleep terrors, occur in the deepest stage of sleep, known as delta sleep or slow wave sleep (SWS). Occurring rarely in adults, the main feature of a night terror is amnesia: that is, remembering nothing or recalling only a brief, frightening image. Sufferers may experience a pressing sensation on the chest or a feeling of invasion, resulting in relatively short episodes of confusion, disorientation, vocal outbursts, and sleepwalking. If you do not wake up a child during a night terror episode, she will likely not remember anything in the morning. It is best to steer children who have gotten up back to bed and they will usually return to sleep within a few minutes. Sleep experts report that people who experience both night terrors and sleepwalking frequently have family histories involving one or the other.

Night terrors are not to be confused with hypnagogic hallucinations. These seemingly bizarre "dreamlets" occur right at the point of falling asleep and involve vivid, startling imagery. They can be frightening, but the sensation is quite different from the acute panic and obscure images associated with night terrors.

Some researchers have suggested that sleepwalking, known in medical terms as "somnambulism," is the culmination of a night terror. Sleepwalking affects young and old alike and seems to be an inherited trait. Since it occurs primarily in the deeper non–REM sleep stages, sleepwalkers rarely talk and do not remember the episode. Still, they can be quite active: walking around, using the bathroom, and so forth. This is potentially dangerous, because the individual lacks the judgment they would usually have when awake. The sleepwalker usually cannot be awakened; if an attempt is made, they will be disoriented and confused. If you wake up to find a family member sleepwalking, you are advised to do the following: steer the sleeper back to bed, protecting them from injury. Don't try to awaken them. The following is a sample of what Mazza recommends to keep a sleepwalker safe:

- keep doors and windows locked; if necessary, install a second, out-of-reach lock for children.
- have the sleepwalker sleep on the first floor of the home or in hotels when traveling.
- when dangerous behavior is associated with sleepwalking, consult a physician specializing in sleep disorders.

Counseling and psychotherapy are recommended as effective strategies for dealing with the underlying emotions contributing to the parasomnias. The benzodiazepine (BZDs) class of drugs may work well to control terrors and sleepwalking since they are found to suppress the deepest stages of sleep, stages three and four, during which terrors and sleepwalking occur. As with any addictive medications, however, it would be wise to first consult your health-care practitioner about the use of benzodiazepines. Sometimes sleepwalkers can find relief in afternoon naps.

Researchers are still not certain what triggers the development of these parasomnias. One finding is that a strong stress component is involved. Sleepwalking, for example, can be a feature of post-traumatic stress disorder (PTSD), and/or exposure to early childhood violence. For this reason, relaxation techniques can be particularly effective in combating night terrors and sleepwalking. Deep breathing, systematic muscle relaxation, hypnosis and/or meditation with soothing imagery—all can help put your mind and body at peace, where stressful disturbances are less likely to take hold. Of course, these techniques also help overcome the dread and tension that contribute to your sleep disturbance problem. Refer to chapters 3 and 4 for directions on specific relaxation and hypnotic techniques.

The most common parasomnia in adults, nightmares, deserves special comment. Nightmares typically occur during a REM cycle of sleep, and since REM periods lengthen and predominate later in the night, it makes sense that nightmares would be more easily remembered than other types of dreams—they are fresher in your mind at waking time. Nightmares also have a different character than dreams that occur at other times in the night cycle. They tend to be more vivid, complex, and full of plots, objects, and characters. You may wake up from nightmares sweating, with heart pounding, and wishing to scream, but unable to.

Sleep experts report that more than 80 percent of adult nightmare sufferers complain about recurring nightmares, and that the dream content is usually fear of attack or death. Occasionally, illness brings on nightmares, but for the most part nightmares occur as a result of anxiety-producing events in your life. As mentioned above, while it is very difficult to awaken people who are experiencing night terrors and/or sleepwalking, you are likely to awaken from a nightmare, realize that you have had one, and stay awake for an average of twenty-five minutes.

The best way to manage nightmares is to do regular "inner" work, that is, working with your emotions through dream work, keeping a journal, meditation, and sharing with trusted others as honestly as possible. Mazza writes that "each time we push away an uncomfortable feeling or hold in the words we need to say, we risk having these issues bubble up in the night in horrific dream images." She also counsels us to think of nightmares as gifts, not as scary punishments. Just as all dreams are gifts, nightmares are windows of opportunity for growth and development.

Dr. Hauri reports that a different type of nightmare occurs in people who suffer from PTSD or daytime panic attacks. With PTSD, sufferers may experience flashbacks or anxiety attacks at the transition point between waking and sleeping (stages one or two). Dr. Hauri recommends that counseling for the daytime problem is more effective than focusing on the nightime events.

In the remainder of this chapter, you will learn to desensitize yourself to the negative anticipation of dreaming. You can also find relief from nightmares by learning to manage your reactions to your dreams with basic dream work techniques and advanced techniques such as lucid dreaming. Studies show that people who are good at recalling their dreams are generally better able to confront their own fears and anxieties, which are major contributors to sleeplessness.

Basic Dream Work Techniques

Exploring the meaning of dreams can be learned by almost anybody with practice. Keep an open mind about the process, even if the steps seem strange or don't seem to make any difference at first. A mere awareness of your dreams and their potentially positive power can help alleviate your dread of sleep and pave the way for fewer troubling nightmares. Dreams don't need to control you; remember that it is you and your brain controlling your dreams. Dream work will just help make that control more conscious.

With dream work, it is possible to plan in advance to deal with a recurring troublesome dream. For example, suppose you identify a certain character or theme that reappears regularly in your dreams. Perhaps this character or theme is frightening, causing you to wake up in a sweat every night it appears. You can actually arm yourself against this dream situation, planting helpful escape routes and even objects in your waking mind through self-talk and meditation. Better yet, you can decide to find out why a troublesome character is visiting you in your dreams, so that you can resolve its threat and sleep peacefully.

One woman, for example, was bothered repeatedly by a hooded figure who emanated a bright and piercing light. The dreamer would wake up in a panic every time the figure appeared, and toss and turn in bed for a long time out of anxiety. She would feel agitated and even embarrassed that this dream figure could be so disturbing. Finally she decided to honestly and intensely explore the dream so that she could see behind it and find relief. Before falling asleep, she repeated these phrases to herself:

I will not be afraid when this dream appears.
I will realize I am in a dream, and choose not to wake up.
I will ask what the hooded figure wants.

In just a few nights, she was able to engage the hooded figure in a dialogue. The dreamer saw the blinding light fade, and watched the figure's robe disintegrate to reveal a kindly old gentleman. Once the fear was gone, she was able to go on to explore the meaning of the old man's presence in her dream. In this case she dissected her dream in two ways: she changed the dream while in it—a lucid dreaming technique—and upon awakening she analyzed the dream with her partner to uncover its hidden meaning.

It works best to share your dream with a partner. It could be your significant other, or roommate, or someone who has agreed to be available to you by telephone. In any case, the person must agree to be a committed listener and to ask these basic questions: Who is in your dream? What happened? When did your dream occur? Where were you in the dream? And perhaps, most important, Why now are you having this dream? What message does this dream hold for you?

It will be useful for you to keep in mind that every part of a dream—the characters, symbols, actions taking place—all represent yourself at some level. After all, it is you conducting the dream. No one else is dreaming it for you, although it can feel like the dream is happening *to* you rather than being created *by* you.

Steps to Dream Work

In *The Dream Sharing Sourcebook,* Phyllis Koch-Sheras and Peter Sheras suggest the three "Rs" of dream work: recalling, recording, and reviewing your dreams. Dream recall, or remembering, improves over time with commitment and practice. They say that "confirmed nonrecallers often begin to recall dreams when they come to see how valuable their nighttime images can be for their relationships and their general well-being." Recording is simply keeping track of your dreams by means of jotting the dream down in a notebook or diary. Reviewing means studying the details of your dream, either by yourself or with your partner.

- Keep a dream journal by your bed and every time you wake up write down as much of the dream as you can remember. Don't worry if you can't recall all of the dream; sometimes just getting into the "feeling" of the dream will trigger recall. Dream fragments may be sufficient to piece together the dream action.

- Practice dream recall. Resolve to remember at least one dream per night.
- Become familiar with your typical dream content. Do certain patterns emerge? People? Things? Keep note of these in your dream journal.
- Think about something specific you would like to change in your dreams. If you have a recurring nightmare, think of something—an object or a plot change—that would help you out of it. Be very specific. A magical ladder might help you out of a locked dream room, for instance, or a penetrating question might stop a monster in its tracks.

Bedtime

Start off with deep breathing when you first go to bed to begin easing tension. Then use your favorite relaxation or meditation technique to become as relaxed and receptive as you can be.

- Tell yourself as you begin to drift off that you will recognize that you are dreaming when it occurs, or that you will vividly remember the dream when you awaken.
- Recall the plot change or the magical device you thought would be helpful in your dream.
- Resolve to take it with you into your dream. Visualize and describe in words the object or the change as you drift off.

When you confront a frightening dream figure, whether while you are asleep or awake, try to engage it in dialogue. It's a good thing to be able to scare a monster away; it's a better thing to find out *why* the monster is bothering you, *who* the monster could be, and what fear in your daily life the monster might represent. Instead of fleeing, talk. Ask in a friendly voice, "Who are you?" or even,

"Who am I?" Try to calm down an angry figure by talking instead of fighting. Listen to what it's saying; ask "What do you mean by that?" If the figure still attacks, stare it in the face and let it know you won't back down. Your goal is to achieve a peaceful reconciliation—and to find out something about the attacker. Since your dream character is really a different part of yourself, the answers you get may give you considerable insight into your own fears and concerns. What's more, once you have demystified or decoded a dream figure, it's less likely to come back and haunt your sleep. The awareness and peace you find will probably carry over into your waking life.

Mazza recommends dream incubation as a way to request a dream on a particular subject or for a solution to a problem. Many people have resolved problems or created solutions by "soaking" on it, or sleeping on it. To incubate, or "hatch," a dream, here are some of the steps she recommends:

- Write your specific question in your dream journal or note-book before going to bed.
- Write your question in the simplest language possible, and be specific.
- Record whatever you remember of a dream when you wake up; no matter what you dream, review it in terms of your question.
- If you want an answer to a question about a certain person, place, or thing, vividly picture it before going to sleep, or gaze at a photo if you have one. Allow yourself to feel any associated feelings, or jot down your feelings in your dream diary.

Advanced Dream Work: Using Lucid Dreaming to Change Your Dreams

Although guiding and controlling dreams was a hallmark of healing for many ancient peoples, the term "lucidity" was not introduced into modern dream work until the early 1900s. But only recently has the technique gained acceptance as a way to control frightening dreams.

As the name suggests, lucid dreaming is a way to make your dreams visible and clear to you: you realize you are in a dream, you decide to change that dream, and you let yourself explore that dream. In regular dreams the dreamers may not be aware that they are dreaming until awakening. That accounts for the power of dreaming: it feels like a real-life experience. In a lucid dream, however, the dreamer can see without waking up that the experience is only a dream. The realization strips the terror from the dream. A lucid dreamer can then enter the dream, take a conscious and active role in it, and direct it away from a frightening or negative ending. He can even choose to explore the dream, turning monsters into insightful characters and nightmares into learning experiences.

It can be exhilarating to realize that you can actually change the course of your dreams. After all, that's just what will free you from the horror of your nightmares: you can turn them into neutral, even positive, dreams. In choosing from the array of options available to you, there are just a few guidelines to keep in mind. For one thing, it's best not to hope to create a perfect dream. You simply want to work within the dream you find yourself in, to steer it in a positive direction. Think about cooperating, not manipulating. Think about controlling your own actions, not the whole dream.

One way to plan your role in a dream is to arm yourself with the tools you'll need in the dream. Spend some time thinking about your typical dream patterns; start keeping a dream journal so you can remember your dreams, and find similarities among them. You don't need to write down every detail, but try to write something every morning so you get used to capturing the experience of dreaming. If you can identify a particular dream or detail that recurs, ask yourself what change you would like to see in it. Think of a specific plot-twist, action, or helpful object you would like to have in your dream. You can then incorporate vivid images of that change into your pre-bed relaxation ritual. You want to fix the image in your head and trigger an association between the beginning of the dream and the change you have planned. Run through a version of your typical dream in your head, focusing on the change you want to insert. A few sentences of self-talk as you drift off can help you take that change with you into your dream. For example, "When the muggers chase me around the corner, a policeman or somebody will be there to help me."

Once you have become lucid in a dream (you realize you *are* in a dream), what will you do? Take action. Reason with the monster to go away; look for the escape ladder you know you planted in the room. This is your opportunity to take control. Instead of hoping to change the entire dreamscape, focus in on your own actions. Chances are that once you respond in an aware way to your dream surroundings, the dream itself will change to accommodate you. Maybe the monster will dissolve; maybe it will become a kind person willing to talk to you. Since you'll know you're dreaming, you'll find many more options available to you, and much less reason to fear the thing that threatens you.

Lucid dreamers report that their dreams take on a particular vividness once they become self-aware in a dream. They also often experience a new sense of freedom—not just from nightmares, but from many constraints and fears of daily life. Some people suffering from phobias have even experienced a decrease in deep-seated waking fears—of heights, say, or dogs—after confronting them in lucid dreams. Of course the technique is not a cure-all for life's problems. Not all your dreams can be lucid, either. About 10 percent of the population dreams lucidly on a regular basis without working on the technique; these people report about one lucid dream per month. Practice with the faith that you can learn to achieve lucid dreaming and summon the experience when needed.

Lucid dreaming does not have to be used exclusively with nightmares. Another dreamer reported using lucidity to simply explore a pleasant but mysterious image of a blond, tall, tan man who kept cropping up in her dreams, smiling. She discovered that the man was her reflection, and that he appeared at times when she felt great amounts of competence and self-esteem. The blond man reinforced her feeling of power, and she would awaken feeling renewed and strong.

What are the signs that lucidity is happening for you? Phyllis Koch-Sheras, Ann Hollier, and Brooke Jones in their book, *Dream On,* suggest that you look for the following cues:

- When you begin examining your dream environment more critically, such as with recognition of characters or objects from previous dreams
- When you begin thinking about your dream symbols and what they mean *while you are dreaming*
- When you begin to look for signs that what you are experiencing is a dream

Be Calmly Persistent

If you feel that these dream work techniques are not working for you, do not succumb to feelings of failure and give up altogether. Learning to experience awareness and control of your dreams is a skill that improves with practice. If you know that bad dreams are disrupting your sleep, summon up the courage to examine your dreams through waking fantasy or lucidity.

Remember that it takes time to achieve the mind-set and level of awareness you need to experience lucid dreaming at will. What's more, even when you've begun to dream lucidly, you might be misled by the idea of "controlling" your dreams completely. It might not work simply to tell the monster to go away. Maybe you need to ask it harder questions, such as, "Are you my mother?" Maybe you need to ask it for help, or simply demonstrate your resolve and courage by staring it in the eyes. The idea is to cooperate with your dreams rather than to control them. You want to control your own behavior rather than the dream content. In this way, you can allow the dream agenda to freely present itself.

Conversing with your dream characters may begin a process of integrating them into your waking life, so that you become less fearful of them and consequently less fearful and anxious while awake. Jayne Gackenbach and Jane Bosveld, in their book *Control Your Dreams,* explain that if you "battle" with dream characters, it may only bury the problem deeper. Ideally, you want to confront your dream fears in a positive way. This serves as a desensitizing process, fortifying you to confront them in your waking life. Dealing directly with your dream conflicts and anxieties in an assertive manner is a sort of "role play" for dealing assertively with difficulties in life. It reminds you that you have the power to reframe the way you see the circumstances you find yourself in— whether awake or asleep. If you choose to practice reframing your dream situations in your unconscious life, you will be building your ability to reframe situations in your waking life.

9

Menopause
and Sleep

There was a time when menopause was a nondiscussable topic. Mothers may have mentioned the "change," but they would not, could not, elaborate. Menopause carried with it a stigma of debilitation, born in part of misinformation. Women suffered in silence, and a major part of that suffering was, and is, sleeplessness.

We can safely say times have changed for the better, and women feel free, out of wisdom and necessity, to ask for what they want. No longer a dark mystery, menopause is considered almost a rite of passage, a positive transition freeing women to embrace the potential of the second half of their lives. This shift in perspective has prompted many excellent books on the subject. To name just a few, Christiane Northrup, MD, *The Wisdom of Menopause;* Joyce Walsleben, Ph.D, *Woman's Guide to Sleep;* and John Lee, MD, *What your Doctor May Not Tell You About Premenopause* provide thorough and practical information about the causes and treatment of menopause. This chapter provides highlights from these and other sources.

Hormone Replacement Therapy (HRT)

What must be mentioned first is what's at the heart of the menopause puzzle: the use of hormone replacement therapy, or HRT.

Thought for decades to decrease the negative effects of menopause and protect against heart disease, new information is rapidly
emerging to prove otherwise. For example, as recently as August
2003, Reuters Health reported that new British research adds to
mounting evidence of the dangers of HRT and confusion about
the benefits versus the risks of taking HRT. These studies support
the results of the highly touted Women's Health Initiative (WHI)
study released in 2002 and reported in the *New England Journal
of Medicine*. In the initial WHI study researchers found that the
hormones investigated (an estrogen and progestin combination)
may in fact increase the risk for heart attacks, stroke, blood clots,
and breast cancer. The American College of Obstetricians and
Gynecologists (ACOG) *Managing Menopause* magazine stated in its
spring/summer 2003 issue that another part of the WHI released
in 2003 challenged the previously held notion that hormone therapy significantly improves a woman's concentration, sleep, sex life,
and overall quality of life.

Nevertheless, some women, after careful consideration with
their health-care professionals, are choosing to stay on hormones
because of the disruptive effects of menopause. A *Washington Post*
article on August 3, 2002, reported, "Because of the increased
risk for heart attacks, stroke, blood clots and breast cancer appears to be relatively low, many doctors say they will put patients
back on hormones as long as they understand the risks, especially
if they have no family history of heart disease or breast cancer."

It is not surprising then, that women are confused and angry
about the state of hormone replacement therapy and menopause. Since the case for HRT use or not seems to change daily,
doubt has definitely been cast on the wisdom of subjecting your
body to possible problems. Yet, the symptoms of menopause can
be debilitating enough that women are forced to weigh the odds,
asking, "Should I risk ill health in the long run for a good night's
sleep in the short run?"

Pat Dougherty, nurse practitioner at the Women's Midlife Center at the University of Virginia, says:

In general, our feeling is that HRT should be prescribed for women who have significantly symptomatic hot flashes/night sweats that impact their quality of life and are not relieved by CAM [complementary and alternative medicine] and lifestyle changes. The shortest duration and lowest effective dose of HRT is prescribed. Since most women are only significantly symptomatic for three to five years, we think HRT is not unreasonable for symptom management in the average woman. In a woman with diagnosed cardiac disease or significant risk factors for cardiac disease (obesity, hypertension, smoker, diabetes, elevated cholesterol) we would shy away from HRT or at least proceed gingerly. A family history of breast cancer itself is not a contraindication to HRT, but a *strong* family history (multiple first and second degree relatives) suggests an inherited genetic mutation for which HRT would be ill-advised.

If a woman chooses CAM, Dougherty cautions the following, which is an opinion echoed throughout medical literature: "Remember that we don't have a lot of safety or efficacy information on many of the alternative methods that are being touted for relief of perimenopausal symptoms, so you have to proceed with caution there as well." She recommends the Web site of the North American Menopause Society (NAMS), for the latest information: www.menopause.org.

Professor Valerie Beral of Britain's Cancer Research UK, who headed the British research team on HRT, sums it up by saying "The risk goes up with the duration of use and is apparent within one to two years." Beral advised women who are confused about taking HRT to consult their doctors, but she added, "There is no simple answer."

Women should beware of anyone making a claim that there is an answer. The doctor will tell you one thing, the herbal specialist another thing, and the clinical nutritionist yet another. In light of this, the specifics of estrogen and progesterone are not discussed. Rather, women are advised to ask their health-care professional(s) for an opinion based on the patient's overall health habits and family history. The following section, however, steers women toward commonly held beliefs about herbal remedies that have stood the test of time, even if they have not been clinically proven to be effective. The recommended herbs do not appear to pose any risk or have any significant side effects.

Menopause exhibits a myriad of symptoms that are discussed in this chapter, with an emphasis on one of menopause's hallmarks: sleeplessness.

Sophie, for example, considered herself a sound sleeper for most of her life, until she hit her late forties and began noticing a change in her sleep quality. She noticed she would awaken between 3 A.M. and 4 A.M. several nights in a row at certain times in the month, sometimes coinciding with her monthly cycle and sometimes in the middle of it. She attributed her sleeplessness to that as well as to a stressful work project, but noticed the same pattern reoccurring when her work stress decreased. Sometimes she was so wide awake she felt like she had just slept a full night and/or had a heavy dose of caffeine.

This chapter presents highlights of the issue and provides information on "what's out there," so that women can make an informed choice that feels right. First, the mechanics of menopause are briefly discussed in light of sleep problems, followed by possible treatment choices, ranging from HRT to CAM. As always, this information should be discussed with health-care provider(s) before taking any action.

Mechanics of Menopause

A woman's hormonal levels are in a state of flux from puberty through menopause. She may notice the changes beginning around her thirties, culminating in actual menopause, or cessation of monthly menstrual cycles. The decline in the body's production of estrogen, especially, is likely the culprit for hot flashes, night sweats, and sleeplessness. The ACOG reports that before menopause, estrogen is secreted in large amounts by the ovaries, and may drop by 75 percent or more after menopause. Estrogen stimulates the production of the brain chemical serotonin, which among many other things, regulates sleep patterns. Less estrogen can mean disrupted sleep. Estrogen also acts as part of the body's natural temperature regulation system. When estrogen levels drop, the surface blood vessels in the skin suddenly dilate, with subsequent increased blood flow to the skin. Called hot flashes or hot flushes, this increased flow triggers the sweat glands to release perspiration. This moisture on the skin's surface rapidly evaporates and causes cooling of the skin.

Hot Flashes/Night Sweats

Bringing extra blood to the skin's surface is the normal way a human body reacts to cause cooling when body temperature rises. But with perimenopause and menopause, this may happen so profusely that a woman can wake up many times during the night, drenched in sweat. She may feel the annoying sensations of her pulse racing and heart beating rapidly.

According to NAMS, hot flashes that occur with drenching perspiration while sleeping are called night sweats. While these events may not be strong enough to cause someone to wake up, the falling estrogen levels alone can disrupt patterns of healthy deep sleep. In its popular and practical *Menopause Guidebook*, NAMS reports,

"While it is a myth that menopause itself makes a woman irritable, inadequate sleep causes fatigue, which may lead to irritability."

Fifty to 75 percent of women report hot flashes during menopause. Some women, however, pass through menopause without many hot flashes at all. There may be genetic, physiologic, environmental, and cultural differences in women, all exerting an influence on how women experience the severity and frequency of hot flashes. Hot flashes can occur at any time of the night or day. A hot flash generally lasts from thirty seconds to thirty minutes, but most last only two to three minutes. Some women report having hot flashes as frequently as once per hour. Other women have hot flashes only occasionally. In one study, 20 percent of women reported daily hot flashes, and almost half of those women rated the severity of those hot flashes as moderate to severe.

Various studies suggest that 25 percent or more of women have sleep disturbances because of hot flashes around the time of menopause. Women over age forty-five report more sleep problems than younger women or men of the same age. These problems can include difficulty falling asleep, which sleep experts call longer latency to sleep onset. Women may also experience frequent nighttime awakenings, also known as lack of sleep continuity or sleep fragmentation. Many women report feeling that they have less deep, restful sleep. This feeling has been supported by sleep studies that have shown less time spent in slow wave sleep (SWS), or deep sleep, also known as delta sleep.

One sleep study demonstrated that physiologic measurements of sleep disturbances coincided with the occurrence of hot flashes and night sweats. The sleep disturbances experienced because of hot flashes can cause sleep deprivation, which shows up the next day as nervousness, irritability, and daytime tiredness.

Two areas of the brain, the hypothalamus and pituitary gland, regulate the amount of circulating estrogen. Estrogen levels are also thought to be under the influence of parts of the brain that control moods and circadian rhythms, and are susceptible to "triggers" such as certain foods, cigarette smoking, and psychological stress. Women who have a previous history of issues with stress and emotions may have more difficulty adjusting to hot flashes and other changes that come with menopause. This may explain why some women hardly notice the coming and going of menopause, while others acutely feel its effects.

What to Do about Night Sweats

NAMS recommends that women:

- Avoid "triggers" such as external heat (e.g., a warm room or use of a hair dryer), hot drinks, hot or spicy foods, alcohol, and caffeine.
- Be aware that some drugs prescribed for cancer chemotherapy such as tamoxifen (Nolvadex) and for prevention or treatment of osteoporosis, raloxifene (Evista), can cause hot flashes.
- Keep cool by dressing in layers, which can be removed as needed.
- Keep cool by sleeping in a cool room and using a fan.
- Reduce stress by using meditation, yoga, biofeedback, visualization, massage, or by taking a leisurely bath.
- Try paced respiration (deep, slow abdominal breathing) when a hot flash is starting during the day or upon awakening from a night sweat.
- Exercise regularly to reduce stress and promote better, more restorative sleep.

Natural Sleep Aids: Soy Isoflavones and Black Cohosh

Soy isoflavones and black cohosh are plant products that have been used here and in Europe for treatment of hot flashes. Soy foods have been used for centuries in Asia, and Asian women have been observed to have fewer problems with hot flashes and other menopausal complaints. A typical traditional Asian diet contains around forty to eighty milligrams of isoflavones per day. Contrast this with the typical North American diet, which contains less than three milligrams of isoflavones per day. One gram of soy protein usually contains about 1.5 milligrams of isoflavones. Manufacturers of soy products such as tofu, tempeh, and miso are beginning to list the amount of isoflavones in their packaged products. The NAMS Web site (see Sources for Additional Information at end of this chapter) contains a useful chart that lists the isoflavone levels in various soy food products. Following a diet that is rich in fruits and vegetables, including soy foods, can also lower serum lipids, help prevent osteoporosis, and provide many other health benefits.

These two botanicals have been studied in clinical trials and have been shown to be effective in reducing hot flashes. There have not been adverse risks reported with either soy derivatives or black cohosh. However, taking isoflavones as supplements may be less effective than eating foods rich in isoflavones, as discussed above. Recent thinking, again not sufficiently studied, is that it is better to eat isoflavones or soy in foods rather than isolate them in supplements.

Isoflavones

These are a type of phytoestrogen, or estrogen derived from plant products. Soy and red clover are common sources of isoflavones. Isoflavones are also found in flaxseed, peanuts, beans, whole grains, and peas. Isoflavones have a mild estrogenic effect and can have a modest effect on hot flashes. Supplemental isoflavone preparations are thought to be generally less effective than whole soy foods in reducing menopausal symptoms. Also, processing of whole soy into food products can destroy some of the isoflavone content. Because of their mild estrogenic effect, isoflavones are not recommended for women who have had breast cancer. Women who are taking tamoxifen, an antiestrogenic medication, may not find isoflavones to be effective.

Black cohosh (*Actaea racemosa*) is a North American plant also known as black snakeroot or bugbane, and can be found under the brand name Remifemin. Black cohosh was the chief botanical extract in Lydia Pinkham's Vegetable Compound, a famous patented medication that was introduced in the late 1800s and promoted as a treatment for a wide range of gynecologic disorders. Black cohosh has been used by Native Americans for generations for various gynecologic complaints, sleep disorders. and depression. Black cohosh is also used extensively in Germany, where it is one of the most commonly used treatments for hot flashes. Because of its estrogenic activity, it is recommended to be used only for less than six months and may have an effect on breast and endometrial tissue. The daily dosage is between twenty and forty milligrams per day to forty-eight to eighty milligrams per day. Improvement in hot flashes is generally seen in two to four weeks. Black cohosh has been used to treat hot flashes for many years in Europe and has not been associated with adverse outcomes. As with isoflavones, black cohosh may not be effective in women who are taking tamoxifen. Side effects of black cohosh supplements may include stomach irritation or low blood pressure.

Other Natural Sleep Aids

Valerian

Valerian root is well known as one of the most effective herbs for insomnia. Ross, Brenner, and Goldberg, authors of the *Alternative Medicine Definitive Guide to Sleep Disorders,* cite a scientific team representing the European community that has reviewed the research available on valerian and concluded that it is a safe nighttime sleep aid. If you are put off by its odor as a tea, take it in extract, tincture, or capsule form, 30–60 minutes before bedtime. Christopher Hobbs writes in *Herbal Remedies for Dummies*, that "the smell alone is enough to put some people out . . . Steep the valerian for 30 minutes in a closed pot, and drink one cup, several times daily." Some herbalists recommend taking valerian for only a month or as needed per situation, as it can be mildly habit-forming. Most sources say, however, that valerian is the herb of choice for treating insomnia, and that it is not addictive and does not produce morning hangover.

Kava Kava

Also known simply as "kava," this herb acts as a natural tranquilizer and can be taken in capsule or tablet form, as a tincture or tea. Herbalists recommend kava for tension, nervousness, tight muscles, and mild depression, as well as insomnia. However, the National Center for Complementary and Alternative Medicine (NCCAM) has recently released a consumer advisory on kava, citing safety as a concern for those people with liver disease or liver problems, or who are taking drugs that can affect the liver (July 23, 2002). Check with your health-care provider before using this herb.

Melatonin

Melatonin is a naturally occurring hormone secreted by the pineal gland in the brain. It controls sleeping and waking cycles and regulates the body's internal time clock or circadian rhythms. While the amount of the hormone produced is based primarily on the body's exposure to light, there are other factors that influence melatonin production, such as aging. While synthetically derived melatonin supplements are considered safe for short term use, its long term effects are unknown. Studies show that it is quick acting (people fall asleep within 30 minutes of taking it), so that it benefits sleep onset latency in stages one and two (light sleep). Melatonin can also increase delta (deep sleep) and REM sleep, which may account for the reason that people report vivid dreams when taking the supplement. There are some caveats for its use with pregnant and nursing mothers and people with severe allergies, among other things, so you would be wise to consult your health care practitioner before using melatonin.

5-HTP

Melatonin is derived from the molecule 5-HTP, or 5-hydroxytryptophan. Considered safe and effective for sleep problems, 5-HTP is also useful for treating symptoms of PMS and seasonal affective disorder (SAD). It can be taken in tablet or capsule form. Consult an herbalist for recommended dosage.

In *The Wisdom of Menopause*, Dr. Northrup says, "Even natural substances such as valerian, natural progesterone, and kava kava may eventually lose their effectiveness over time, because they bind to the same place in the brain as prescription sleep drugs. It's best to use them sparingly, and only after you've tried other routes to a good night's sleep."

Soy and Vitamin E

Dr. Andrew Weil in his *Self Healing Newsletter* suggests eating foods containing soy and vitamin E to cope with hot flashes and insomnia. Soy provides a gentle estrogenic effect on the body and may also help build bones and reduce the risk of breast cancer. Foods rich in soy are tofu, soy milk, green soybeans, and some meat substitutes.

Dr. Weil also comments that it can be difficult to get optimum amounts of vitamin E from food alone, especially if you are eating a low-fat diet. He suggests taking a vitamin E supplement, because to obtain the minimum daily dose he recommends you would have to consume a pound of sunflower seeds or more than five pounds of wheat germ!

Dr. Hauri warns: "If you decide to try any herbal preparation, we suggest that you work with someone who is an expert in herbs, since overdoses of herbs or the wrong combinations, as with any substance, can cause serious side effects, especially if you combine them with certain prescription drugs."

Exercise

Exercise is a wonderful way to deal with the sleeplessness of menopause. Regular, aerobic exercise causes the body to release endorphins, the body's natural opioids. These "feel good" hormones can promote an overall sense of well-being, decrease stress and anxiety, and can help support better sleep. Many women find that regular exercise also reduces the frequency and severity of hot flashes. Women should avoid strenuous exercise just before bedtime, and leave at least two to three hours between exercise and bedtime.

Avoiding cigarettes is another helpful way to combat hot flashes. Smoking cigarettes has been shown to decrease the amount of circulating estrogens in a woman's body and can alter estrogen metabolism by several different mechanisms. It has been observed that women who smoke cigarettes experience menopause one to two years earlier than women who don't smoke. This phenomenon is thought to occur because the chemicals in cigarette smoke destroy the cells within the ovary that produce estrogen. Clinical trials have shown that women who smoke have an increased rate of moderate to severe hot flashes that correlates with the number of cigarettes smoked per day and the number of years of cigarette use.

A Final Note

In the past, menopause was often viewed with trepidation by many women and was a topic simply avoided by many heath-care practitioners. Today, however, much more information is available directly to women through the media and, more recently, the internet. Conventional health-care practitioners as well as practitioners of CAM are recognizing the need to better inform women about the process of menopause and offer therapies to ease the symptoms of this natural transitional period. Today women can choose from a wide variety of pharmacologic medications and herbal supplements to help ease the symptoms of menopause. Each has its own set of drawbacks. Cost, side effects, and possible interactions with other medications should all be taken into consideration. After conferring with a health-care practitioner, a woman may want to consider stopping any unnecessary medications and supplements. In this way she can experience her "baseline" hormonal status. Then, if she wishes, she can gradually reintroduce measures such as soy in the diet or black cohosh supplements to see what works best. Remember, what is best for each individual is an informed choice based on experience and learning.

Menopause is now regarded as a natural phase of a woman's life, not a disease process. Thankfully, much has been written to take the fear and dread out of this natural changeover. It is, after all, an inevitable process, one that women can choose to view as an evolutionary gift rather than a curse. Chinese herbal medicine practitioners have a combination of herbs called "Joyful Change" designed for menopause. Dr. Lee and Dr. Hanley refer to menopause as a life cycle to be respected and looked forward to and that it was once called the "dangerous age" because so many women begin speaking their minds at this time of life. The doctors go on to say, "What the world needs more than anything is for a woman to have the courage to speak her mind."

Sources for Additional Information

American College of Obstetricians and Gynecologists (ACOG)
http://www.acog.org
P.O. Box 96920
Washington, D.C. 20090

ConsumerLab
http://www.consumerlab.com
ConsumerLab.com, LLC
333 Mamaroneck Avenue
White Plains, NY 10605
(914) 722-9149
(This is a commercial Web site that provides information for
   a fee.)

iVillage Women's Health
http://www.ivillagehealth.com

National Association for Women's Health (NAWH)
http://www.nawh.org
300 West Adams, Suite 328
Chicago, IL 60606
(312) 786-1468

National Sleep Foundation (NSF)
http://www.sleepfoundation.org
1522 K Street NW, Suite 500
Washington, D.C. 20005

National Women's Health Resource Center
http://www.healthywomen.org
120 Albany Street, Suite 820
New Brunswick, NJ 08901
(877) 986-9472

North American Menopause Society (NAMS)
http://www.menopause.org
P.O. Box 94527
Cleveland, OH 44101
(800) 774-5341

The American Botanical Council
http://www.herbalgram.org
6200 Manor Road
Austin, TX 78723
(512) 926-4900
(This is a commercial Web site that provides information for a
   fee.)

The National Center for Complementary and Alternative Medicine
   (NCCAM)
http://nccam.nih.gov

The National Institutes of Health
Office of Dietary Supplements
http://dietary-supplements.info.nih.gov

The National Library of Medicine
http://www.nlm.nih.gov

10

Aging and Sleep

First, who is considered "elderly?" In nineteenth-century Germany, Bismarck defined sixty-five as the age at which a person would be eligible for social security. Considering the average life span was forty-six years at that time, the state would not have had to support many people! Now the average life span in developed countries is seventy-six—and the fastest growing segment of the older population is that of those over age eighty-five! According to an article from the Centers for Disease Control on public health and aging, in the United States alone, the number of people at or over eighty years of age is expected to increase from 9.3 million in 2000 to 19.5 million in 2030.

Medicare and the field of gerontology adopted sixty-five as the defining age for elderly people in this country, despite the American Association for Retired Persons (AARP) definition. AARP considers people at fifty to be part of their organization and "mature," and many discount plans use the benchmark age of fifty-five for "senior" programs. It is clear that because of the burgeoning growth of this segment of the population, a general redefinition of the word "elderly," is in order. In the meantime, for the purposes of this chapter, people age sixty-five and greater will be considered "elderly," as this is what is used as a starting point for medical studies.

Specifics about Sleep and Aging

Why the quality of our sleep changes as we age is not entirely understood physiologically. However, there are many confounding factors, such as gender and the environment, which may help to explain the lighter, more fragmented sleep in the elderly. For example, elderly women are twice as likely as men to complain of persistent insomnia, which may be related to postmenopausal hormonal changes. Insomnia is more common in older African American women, people with depression, and those with chronic illness. The pain from chronic illness or acute disease may keep people from falling asleep, anxiety and resulting obsessive thoughts may wake them up, and needing to urinate may also contribute to early morning awakening.

Approximately two thirds of elderly people in nursing homes have sleep problems. Understandably the transition from home independence to institutional dependence can create feelings of frustration in many residents, inhibiting their sleep. Their bed is unfamiliar, lighting is brighter, noise is louder, and privacy has decreased or disappeared altogether.

Published reports from studies include the following statistics:

For those over sixty-five, the greatest problem with sleep is difficulty falling asleep (37 percent), nighttime awakening (29 percent), and early morning awakening (19 percent). Sleep apnea, periodic leg movement disorder, restless legs, and narcolepsy are the main sleep disorders that increase in incidence with age. Therefore, it is difficult to say if the awakenings are due to age or to other conditions (see below under Medical Evaluation). It is not true that elderly people need less sleep than their younger counterparts. It is true, however, that sleep loss of as little as 1½ hours in a night can result in up to 33 percent less alertness during the next day for all of us.

The Stages of Sleep

As we discussed in detail in chapter 1, there are two "states" of sleep and four "stages." The two states are REM and NREM. REM sleep is that of an activated brain. NREM is that of a quiescent brain. The four stages occur in NREM sleep. Stages one and two are lighter sleep when sleep begins. Stages three and four are deeper sleep, also called delta wave sleep. Overall, the elderly have less continuity in their sleep, that is, their sleep does not progress evenly throughout the stages, meaning they frequently awaken during the night. For example, there is an earlier onset of REM sleep and a decrease in the total amount of REM sleep. Even as early as age twenty, the amount of time spent in stages three and four decreases, so that by age ninety, these stages may disappear entirely, meaning sleep is lighter and perhaps less restful.

The sleep-wake cycle is also changed in the elderly. Older people tend to have what is termed as "advanced sleep phase syndrome" (ASPS), in which they fall asleep early and awaken early. Disturbances to the cycle may be affected by such things as travel across time zones, shift work and sleep deprivation, all less tolerated by older people. In addition, older people are more easily awakened by noise than younger people. This is certainly an additional factor in institutional settings such as nursing homes and hospitals, which may be noisier than a home environment. There also may be less natural light exposure in those settings.

Dementia represents a special case in the elderly, with more associated sleep problems than with normal aging. Demented individuals take longer to get to sleep, have more frequent awakenings, are more active when awakened, and sleep more during the day. Sometimes there is a day/night sleep reversal, meaning they shift their sleeping time from night to day. Unfortunately about 50 percent of people over the age of eighty-five have some degree of dementia. Variations of dementia appear as Alzheimer's, ministrokes, or dementia associated with Parkinson's.

Primary Sleep Disorders

Sleep apnea is one of the most common sleep disorders. Estimates of the prevalence of this disorder range from 26 percent to 73 percent of the elderly population. What happens is that breathing stops, oxygen levels drop, the person wakes up briefly, gasps for breath, goes back to sleep for awhile, and the cycle starts again. Sleep apnea is more common in men than in women and is seen more often in obese people than in thin people. It is characterized in the elderly as much as in younger people by snoring and excessive daytime sleepiness. We joke about snoring, but sleep apnea can lead to serious medical problems and should not be taken lightly. These include life-threatening cardiac rhythm problems (heart beats either too fast or too slow), heart attacks, coronary artery disease, strokes, high blood pressure, and memory problems. Motor vehicle accidents due to drowsiness are more common in people with sleep apnea than in other individuals. Read more about sleep apnea in chapter 12, "Sleep Disorders."

Periodic Limb Movement Disorder (PLM) involves repetitive movements of the legs every twenty to forty seconds during NREM sleep. This tends to be in the lighter sleep stages. The incidence of this increases with age, and, according to one study, is found in one third of community-dwelling elderly. There is also an increased incidence in people with Parkinson's disease, kidney disease, and diabetes.

Restless Legs Syndrome (RLS), despite its name, can involve arms as well as legs. This occurs particularly on retiring but can occur during the day as well. It is a continuous movement, not intermittent like PLM. Patients complain of a crawling sensation within their limbs. Moving the limbs relieves the unpleasant feeling. It can be associated with iron deficiency, dialysis, peripheral neuropathy (painful or tingling sensations in hands and feet), caffeine use, antihistamines (like Benedryl), and some antidepressant medications.

REM Sleep Disorder (also known as REM Behavior Disorder or RBD) was first described in 1985 and is uncommon. It occurs during REM sleep when the person actually acts out a dream sequence. People sometimes yell, talk, and/or hit a bed partner. Lack of muscle tone usually characterizes REM sleep, so this is quite a deviation from normal sleep patterns. More than 90 percent of the patients are male. Usual onset is after age fifty.

Narcolepsy is characterized by (1) persistent drowsiness and falling asleep for no obvious reason in the daytime, (2) cataplexy or sudden loss of muscle tone in response to strong positive or negative emotion, sometimes resulting in slumping to the floor, (3) sleep paralysis, and (4) hypnagogic hallucinations, which are hallucinations reported when first falling asleep; they are similar to very vivid and frightening dreams.

Evaluation: The History

If you are evaluated by your physician for sleep disorders, you will typically be asked the following questions based on the National Institute of Health's guidelines (NIH Consensus Statement on the Treatment of Sleep Disorder of Older People):

1. Are you satisfied with your sleep?
2. Does your bed partner complain of your snoring, having interrupted breathing, or leg movements?
3. Does sleep or fatigue interfere with daytime activities?
   You should establish the duration of the problem. Insomnia lasting less than a week is "transient"; that lasting a few weeks is "short term," and both are usually situational.

4. The next step would be for you *and* your bed partner to fill out a sleep log (diary). You can find an example of a sleep diary in chapter 2.

Medical Evaluation: More Reasons Why Older People Have Sleep Problems

A physical examination should include looking for all the medical problems that could interfere with sleep. The most common of these is arthritis. A Gallup poll conducted by the NSF in 2003 found that 60 percent of people over age fifty who had pain at night interfering with their sleep had arthritis. Sleeping on a painful hip, back, or shoulder is no fun! Many people have either painful or annoying tingling in their hands and feet (paresthesias), which can disturb sleep. Heart and lung problems can cause shortness of breath when the person is in a recumbent position. This includes such diseases as emphysema, chronic bronchitis, and congestive heart failure. Acid indigestion (reflux), common in the elderly, can interfere with sleep. Many medications can get in the way of sleep. Fluid pills (diuretics) can cause increased urination, therefore increasing the need to get up and go to the bathroom. Caffeine-containing medications (some headache pills), steroids (like prednisone), and some inhalers for asthma or bronchitis can cause overstimulation and, therefore, problems with sleep. Some antidepressants, Parkinson's disease medications, and antihypertension medications can cause nightmares. Use of alcohol as a sedative is a problem as the quieting effect wears off after about three to four hours and then there can actually be a stimulant or "miniwithdrawal" effect. Alcohol also worsens sleep apnea.

Nighttime urination is a big factor for many elderly because of kidney disease, diabetes, prostate disease, and congestive heart failure. Diabetes may cause times of excess urination because when blood sugar level is high the person drinks more and thus needs to eliminate more. With prostate enlargement (common in older men) the pressure on the bladder results in more frequent visits to the bathroom during the night, because men feel like they have to go. With congestive heart failure, the supine (back flat, lying face up) position causes nighttime urination.

About 50 percent of insomnia in elderly people is related to psychiatric issues. The principal problems are those of depression, bereavement, and anxiety. Depression, found in about 25 percent of all elderly, is characterized by early morning awakening. Anxiety disorder is usually manifested by difficulty getting to sleep. Loss of usual pleasurable activities or hobbies due to illness, personal losses, and relocation to a new community may all be factors causing depression and anxiety in older people. The good news is that depression is just as treatable in older people as it is in younger people. Some combination of counseling, behavioral changes such as exercise, and the appropriate antidepressant, all do well to treat depression.

Sleep Study (Polysomnography)

A sleep study should be carried out when the doctor suspects a primary sleep disorder, that is, sleep apnea, PLM, Restless Legs Syndrome, or REM sleep disorder. It involves an overnight stay at the sleep lab where the patient is monitored for breathing patterns, brain waves, and muscle movements. Most insurance companies, including Medicare, will pay for this study when ordered by a physician. For a detailed description of what's involved in a sleep study, see chapter 11.

Treatment of Insomnia: The Issue of Medications

Treatment for older people is quite similar to treatment for younger individuals, with one exception—medications need to be much more closely analyzed. First and foremost, the treatment is behavioral; for example, diet, exercise, sleep hygiene, and pre-bed habits, as described in previous chapters. Additionally, Continuous Positive Airway Pressure (CPAP) described in chapter 12 is a device well tolerated by older people. This is good, because surgery is somewhat less successful for sleep apnea in older people. If medications are used, there *must* be much more attention to side effects, doses, drug-drug interaction, and drug-disease interactions.

Medications in general are certainly tricky to manage in older people. There is a wide range of education in the field concerning prescription of medication; some doctors have had geriatric training and some have not. Be persistent about bringing up the following points with your doctor or health-care practitioner. If that person avoids discussing these things with you, then find someone who will. Here's what you should discuss with your physician about medications:

1. You want your doctor to start low, go slow with the dose
2. You want to evaluate the continuing need for the drug
3. You want to be told of any interactions with all other medications
4. Even in thin elderly people, there is proportionately less muscle and more fat; therefore, drugs that are fat soluble will be in the system longer
5. Diseases such as those affecting the kidney, liver, or brain have an impact on the efficacy and/or the side effects of the drug

Chapter 13 describes many commonly used sleep medications, including specific comments about use in the older population. Particularly, the elderly should avoid sleep medications that are long acting. Not everything over the counter is safe. For example, diphenhydramine (trade name Benadryl), found in many over-the-counter sleep remedies, can last more than ten hours, can interfere with alertness, and can cause confusion, dry mouth, constipation, and blurring of vision. Many older people have these conditions to begin with; this drug can worsen preexisting conditions.

In summary, sleep patterns are somewhat different in older people, but the main point to remember is that it is most likely *not* age alone that is causing the problem. Your environment, daytime and pre-bed behaviors, emotional state of mind, and medical history can all contribute to difficulty with sleep, and need to be carefully examined by both you and your doctor or health-care provider. If you don't know where to start, begin by filling out the sleep diary for at least a week. Then you can share this information first with someone you trust, if that makes you feel more comfortable, and then with your doctor. Be honest and diligent about shifting through all the facts contributing to your sleep problem. Sit down and drink one of the herbal teas recommended in chapter 14. You may not find a quick fix for your problem, but rest assured that with calm persistence and belief in yourself, you will find a way to manage your sleep problem. For more on the subject, a good reference is Mark E. Williams, MD, *Complete Guide to Aging and Health* (New York: American Geriatrics Society and Crown Publishing, 1995).

11

Chronic Pain and Sleep

Insomnia and Chronic Illness

Sleep is often one of the first casualties of physical ailments. Not surprisingly, insomnia is one of the most widespread complaints among patients with chronic medical illnesses and particularly in those with pain-related conditions. In fact, pain and insomnia are respectively the two most prevalent health complaints brought to the attention of health professionals. While 58 percent of adults experience symptoms of insomnia a few nights a week, more than half of those suffering from chronic pain conditions describe themselves as "poor sleepers" (2002 National Sleep Foundation Sleep in America Poll). For many people, therefore, chronic pain means chronic sleep disturbances. Problems falling asleep, frequent wakings in the middle of the night, and premature awakening in the morning are the most common sleep problems. Tossing and turning all night along with bouts of light interrupted sleep further trouble many chronic pain sufferers.

Many chronic illnesses, particularly the pain syndromes, can impair sleep. Disturbed sleep is especially frequent in people suffering from arthritis, osteoporosis, fibrositis, low-back pain, temporo-mandibular joint dysfunction, and headaches to name a few. It is also a common problem associated with chronic illnesses such as cancer and diabetes as well as with renal, cardiovascular, and chronic obstructive pulmonary diseases. Acute illness or injury can cause temporary sleep disturbances as it runs its natural course. Many treatments, either medical or surgical, can also trigger sleep problems as a secondary effect. For example, insomnia is almost always associated with the emotional distress that comes before a stressful medical procedure. Clearly, sleep problems associated with chronic pain and illness are widespread and their impact on one's waking life can be very detrimental.

Consequences of Sleep Disturbances

Difficulty sleeping in and of itself can have adverse effects on the quality of one's life. Daytime fatigue, lower energy, mood disturbances, and diminished performance represent only a few of these by-products. Learning to cope with a sleep problem is made even more difficult, however, when it occurs along with medical conditions such as chronic pain or other chronic illnesses. Pain, sleep, and the quality of daytime functioning (emotional well-being, productivity, cognitive abilities) are all interrelated. When both pain and sleep problems occur together, the negative effects on daytime functioning may be more severe than the sum of the individual problems. For example, pain patients who also experience poor sleep report more mood problems and impairment in their daytime activities than people suffering from pain without accompanying insomnia.

Sleep Disturbances, Pain, and Daytime Functioning

An important implication of the interrelated nature of pain, sleep, and daytime functioning is that this relationship can go in more than one direction. For example, not only can pain and sleep problems combine to affect daytime functioning adversely, but the cause and effect relationships can move around the circle in the other direction as well. People who do not get a good night's sleep will often find their pain more intense and unpleasant and have more difficulty coping with their medical condition during the day. Similarly, negative daytime events such as stressful emotional experiences can interfere with sleep, which in turn may lower pain tolerance.

Fortunately, this vicious cycle can be short-circuited to allow people with chronic pain or illness to get the nightly sleep they need. This chapter describes self-management techniques that can help you find more effective methods for coping with sleep disturbances. As a result of better sleep, daytime functioning and the general quality of life often improve as well.

Origins of Sleep Disturbances

Insomnia and Hospitalization

Sometimes a transient sleep problem that seems to be caused by a situational stressor does not resolve itself and develops into a full-fledged case of chronic insomnia. People suffering from chronic pain and other chronic illnesses are especially vulnerable to this type of progression in their sleep problems, particularly if they are hospitalized. Disruption of the sleep cycle in hospitalized patients is routine; not surprisingly then, insomnia is one of the most frequent complaints of hospital patients. Of course, acute pain is a common cause of insomnia in this setting, but there are many other factors affecting hospitalized patients that may lead to the development of persisting sleep problems following discharge.

Hospitals are very noisy environments and patients may be inadvertently awakened at night by roommates, staff, noisy equipment, radio and TV, lights, and more. In addition, patients are often deliberately awakened by staff for a variety of scheduled procedures (e.g., blood samples, medications, etc.) that must be performed at fixed intervals. People often compensate for night-time awakenings with daytime napping. On a short-term basis, this is a very useful strategy. In the long run, however, routine daytime napping can be detrimental to a good night's sleep because napping disrupts the natural sleep-wake cycle of the body. When nighttime awakening due to noise or medical procedures is no longer a problem, sleeping during the day will make it difficult to sleep at night.

Hospitalization may also be associated with emotional distress including anxiety, depression, and feelings of helplessness, all of which can inhibit your ability to sleep. A patient who comes to associate the bed with anxiety and discomfort may have difficulty sleeping in bed long after discharge. This "conditioned insomnia" is worsened by the unhealthy sleep habits often acquired in the hospital. When you are confined to a hospital bed, you begin to associate the bed with many daytime activities (e.g., eating, reading, writing letters) that are incompatible with sleeping. Therefore, the bed becomes your cue for arousal and wakefulness rather than the usual cue for relaxation and rest. Continued use of the bed for activities incompatible with sleep makes it increasingly difficult for you to fall asleep in bed when you want to. (See chapter 5 for more on reconditioning insomnia.)

Pain Behaviors Interfering with Sleep

Even without the stressful experience of hospitalization, you can also condition yourself into similarly poor sleep habits without even realizing it. Chronic pain sufferers often develop methods for coping with the discomfort of pain or with its associated physical limitations. While these pain coping strategies allow you to get through your days, they can also have long-term detrimental effects on your sleep pattern.

Bed rest is the most common method used to alleviate pain. Spending excessive amounts of time lying down attempting to relax, rest, nap, or simply find a comfortable body position may interfere with nighttime sleep. Although bed rest is often recommended and does provide needed rest in the short term, too much time spent in bed may yield undesirable effects. It usually leads to fragmented rather than continuous sleep and prevents healthy rest in the long run.

Using the bed or bedroom as the center of your universe is another natural but detrimental way of coping with physical limitations associated with pain-related conditions. Some people organize their entire daily activities around their bedrooms. Eating, reading, watching TV, paying the bills, and talking on the phone are just a few examples of sleep incompatible activities. The problem is that when you engage regularly in these activities in your bedroom, the bedroom environment becomes associated with wakefulness rather than with sleepiness.

Sleeping late in the morning or making up an extra hour of sleep whenever you have the chance is also likely to cause problems when it becomes habitual. The incidental sleep may provide a temporary escape from the unpleasant experience of pain. You may even feel refreshed after an extra hour of sleep. But taking naps and maintaining an irregular sleep schedule will disrupt your body's natural rhythm and worsen your nighttime sleep pattern.

The important point to remember is that even though pain, illness, or the psychological stress surrounding hospitalization may have been the main factor initially causing your insomnia, there are several behavioral factors currently maintaining your sleep problem. Although most of these behavior patterns are effective and often the only viable alternative in the short term (e.g., bed rest for acute pain), they exacerbate sleep disturbances in the long run. As much as possible, then, you need to take measures to:

1. Avoid prolonged bed rest.
2. Curtail nonsleeping activities in the bedroom.
3. Stay on a regular schedule, avoid naps, and get up at a regular time.

Now that you know what can disrupt your sleep, you can evaluate the nature, time course, and severity of your sleep problem.

Evaluation of Sleep Disorders

Sleep Diary Monitoring

Keeping track of your sleep habits is an important part of gaining a better understanding of your sleep problem. Make several copies of the sleep diary at the end of chapter 2 and try monitoring your sleep pattern for at least one week. Fill in answers each morning, as part of your daily routine.

Maintaining a daily sleep diary serves several purposes. First, it helps you evaluate the severity of your sleep problem. You may realize after a few days of self-monitoring that you get more sleep than you initially thought. This increased awareness may reduce your anxiety and consequently alleviate your sleep problem. If not, establishing a baseline gives you some perspective on your initial problem as you progress through the treatment plan. As sleep improves, some people tend to lose track of how poor it was before treatment and therefore do not realize how much progress they have made.

Keeping a sleep diary also provides you with a better understanding of how your sleep patterns change over time. There may be great night-to-night variations in your sleep pattern; that is, in fact, more the rule than the exception. The sleep diary can also help pinpoint factors that lead to poor sleep and those that are more conducive to a good night's sleep. Finally, the sleep diary is an excellent tool for monitoring your progress throughout treatment. For all these reasons, it's a good idea to apply yourself conscientiously as you embark upon your sleep management program.

Sleep Laboratory Evaluation

Should you be evaluated in a sleep clinic? An overnight sleep evaluation can be a valuable experience, providing you with the most comprehensive assessment of your sleep disorder. The sleep test, called a polysomnogram, can yield valuable information for those suffering from pain and insomnia. It is an essential test for diagnosing several sleep disorders such as sleep apnea, narcolepsy, or periodic leg movements during sleep (see chapter 12 for more information about these disorders).

Before you are scheduled for an overnight sleep evaluation, you will be asked to keep a sleep diary for one to two weeks. You'll then review your diary with a sleep specialist (a psychologist, physician, or both). Your detailed sleep history will be reviewed along with information pertaining to your current sleep-wake schedule, physical problems, medication/substance use, and psychological status. This information helps establish a preliminary diagnosis and initial recommendations and guides the clinician in deciding whether an overnight evaluation is warranted.

Sleep clinics have several private bedrooms available for overnight evaluations. Special care is taken for these bedrooms to look like hotel rooms (with TV and private bathroom) rather than hospital rooms. It is important to provide an environment as much like home as possible. On the night of the evaluation, you arrive at the clinic two hours before your usual bedtime. A sleep technician prepares you for the sleep test. Small electrodes (sensors) are attached to the head and skin so that sleep, respiration, heart rate, and leg movements can be monitored continuously throughout the night. You go to bed at your usual bedtime in a private bedroom. The technician monitors your sleep from an adjacent control room. This sleep evaluation is noninvasive and there is nothing painful to worry about. While you may wonder how you can sleep under such conditions, people can move around almost as freely as if they were sleeping at home without any equipment. It may take longer to fall asleep because you are in a strange environment, but some insomniacs actually fall asleep more quickly because the cues that keep them awake at home are not present in the sleep laboratory. If you need to go to the bathroom during the sleep study, you can call the technician via an intercom and the test is easily interrupted momentarily. The sleep study lasts only as long as your typical night's sleep at home. The technician wakes you up at your usual rising time. After the study is completed, it takes just a few minutes to remove the electrodes and you are ready to return home or go to work.

A one-night polysomnogram will generate about one thousand pages of paper. This data is scored by a sleep technician and used to document how much time was spent in the different stages of sleep as well as any abnormalities in respiration and leg movements. The results are analyzed by a sleep specialist who then reviews the test results with you and makes appropriate treatment recommendations.

When should you have a sleep test? There are several reasons why you might want to undergo an overnight sleep evaluation. For example, if you wake up with cramps in your calves at night, or your bed partner has noted leg jerks during your sleep, you may suffer from Periodic Limb Movement Disorder (PLM) during sleep. As your leg twitches, you may wake up repetitively at night without remembering it on the following day. This condition, formally called nocturnal myoclonus, can either cause problems maintaining sleep at night or impair your ability to stay awake during the day. It is often accompanied by restless legs at bedtime (Restless Leg Syndrome, or RLS). PLM is a common problem in people suffering from chronic pain and particularly in those whose pain radiates to the lower extremities. It is also common in those with chronic illnesses such as renal diseases and in medical conditions causing poor blood circulation (e.g., diabetes).

If you are sleepy during the day, you are overweight, you snore, and your bed partner has noticed pauses in your breathing during sleep, this may be an indication that you have sleep apnea—a breathing disorder occurring during sleep. Sleepers with apnea may stop breathing two to three hundred times in a single night, yet be unaware of it. The most direct consequence of sleep apnea is chronic sleep fragmentation, which leads to severe difficulties staying awake during the day. Complications can also arise from continued interruption in air intake. Sleep apnea is particularly frequent in middle-aged men. You'll find more about it and other disorders in chapter 12.

If, after diligently following the treatment program described in this chapter, you still have problems sleeping at night, it may be because you are unaware of some other sleep disorders that can only be detected by an overnight sleep evaluation.

Pain and Sleep Physiology

Polysomnography has enhanced our understanding of sleep disturbances associated with chronic pain. In pain-free individuals, alpha rhythms, a particular brainwave pattern associated with a mental state of relaxed wakefulness, occur just before sleep onset and are relatively infrequent during sleep. In pain sufferers, however, alpha brainwaves tend to persist into their sleep and particularly into delta, or deep, sleep. As a result of this intrusion, sleep quality is greatly reduced. Because deep sleep is constantly interspersed with this alpha rhythm throughout the night, the patient gets up in the morning with muscle aching, stiffness, and the feeling of having spent the entire night in a constant light sleep without ever having achieved deep sleep. These physiological features of sleep affect pain perception: a high proportion of alpha waves during sleep is associated with an increase in pain sensation and a decrease in energy level. Conversely, a greater amount of delta waves (deep sleep) without alpha intrusion is associated with a decrease in pain intensity and an increase in energy level. Recent research has shown that pain can be induced in people who are otherwise pain free by selectively depriving them of deep sleep. These people wake up in the morning reporting muscle aching and stiffness—reproducing symptoms similar to fibrositis. Clinically this phenomena of alpha-delta sleep has been observed in other pain-related conditions as well, for example arthritis and low-back pain.

Coping Strategies for Overcoming Insomnia

Most treatment methods described earlier in this book can help improve your sleep pattern. In this section, self-management skills specifically designed for patients suffering from chronic pain and sleep disturbances are presented. The ultimate goal of this self-management program is to help you regain control over your sleep patterns. It may not completely cure your insomnia, but it can help you cope more effectively with the occasional poor night's sleep almost everyone experiences once in a while. The two main components to this treatment involve (a) changing maladaptive sleep *habits,* and (b) rethinking your *beliefs* and attitudes about sleeplessness.

Changing Poor Sleep Habits

By now you are probably aware of several unhealthy habits that may interfere with your sleep. Maintaining irregular sleep schedules, napping, spending excessive amount of time in bed, and using the bed/bedroom for nonsleeping activities are the most common maladaptive coping strategies used by those suffering from insomnia and pain. The first part of this program consists of breaking these poor behavior patterns disrupting your sleep.

Go to bed only when sleepy. There is no reason for going to bed if you are not sleepy. It only gives you more time to worry about your inability to sleep and reinforces the negative associations between the bedroom surroundings and sleeplessness.

Get out of bed if you can't sleep. When you are unable to fall asleep or return to sleep in about fifteen minutes, go to another room and engage in some quiet activity. Do not sleep on the couch. Return to bed only when sleepy. Repeat this step as often as necessary throughout the night. Consistent adherence to this regimen will help reassociate your bed/bedroom with getting to sleep quickly. (Chapter 15 offers ideas for appropriate late night activities.)

Maintain a regular rising time. Set the alarm clock and get out of bed at the same time every morning (weekdays and weekends) regardless of the amount of sleep obtained the previous night. Although it may be tempting to stay in bed later because you didn't sleep well the night before, try to maintain a steady sleep-wake schedule. It helps regulate your internal biological clock and synchronize your sleep-wake rhythm.

Use the bed or bedroom for sleep only. Do not read, eat, watch TV, work, or worry in your bed/bedroom either during the day or at night. Sex is the only exception to this rule. By curtailing nonsleeping activities in the bed/bedroom, it will strengthen the cuing properties of this environment for sleep. Just as you may have developed strong associations between the kitchen and hunger or between a particular chair and relaxation, you want to reinforce the associations between your bedroom and sleep.

Avoid daytime napping. When you stay awake all day, you are sleepier at night. If a nap is unavoidable, limit it to one hour per day and schedule it before 3 P.M. in order to minimize interference with nighttime sleep.

Allow yourself at least one hour before bedtime to unwind. Use this transitional period to engage in your pre-bedtime rituals (e.g., reading, bathing, brushing teeth, etc.). Do not rehash events of the day or plan tomorrow's schedule. Schedule another time during the day or early evening to do problem solving and to write down worries and concerns. After a sleepless night, minimize problem solving on the following day as everything will seem more complicated or more difficult to handle than it really is.

Sleep Restriction

Bed rest is the most common strategy used to cope with both pain and sleep disturbances. While it is an effective and sometimes the only alternative method of dealing with acute pain and sleep problems, excessive amounts of time spent in bed may disrupt sleep patterns. Even though you may get the impression that at least you're getting some rest, too much time lying down awake will worsen rather than improve your sleep pattern. Sleep restriction is a somewhat paradoxical method of treating chronic insomnia. This treatment method was designed by Art Spielman, a psychologist at City College of New York, and consists of curtailing the amount of time spent in bed to the actual amount of sleep you get. You need first to determine how much time per night you typically spend in bed and how much of that time is spent asleep. Then you curtail your time in bed to the actual amount of sleep. Here is how it works. After you have kept a sleep diary for one week, calculate your nightly average of (a) total sleep time, (b) time spent in bed, and (c) sleep efficiency:

$$\frac{\text{Total Sleep Time} \times 100}{\text{Time in Bed}} = \text{Sleep Efficiency}$$

For example, if you were getting an average of six hours of sleep per night out of nine hours spent in bed, your sleep efficiency would be 66.7 percent. Your task is then to restrict the amount of time you spend in bed to the actual amount of sleep. In this example, you would initially restrict your time in bed to six hours per night. This is your "sleep window" for the first week of treatment. As your sleep improves, you gradually extend time in bed by adding twenty to thirty minutes to your sleep window every week. As long as your sleep efficiency is greater than 85 percent, you continue increasing time in bed until you reach an optimal sleep duration. If your sleep efficiency falls below 80 percent, you should decrease time in bed by twenty to thirty minutes for the following week. When sleep efficiency falls between 80 percent and 85 percent you simply maintain the same time in bed for an additional week. This sleep restriction procedure will help consolidate your sleep at night. Initially, you may feel sleepier during the day; don't worry, this is normal. Because you will be sleep deprived, you will also fall asleep faster and sleep more deeply at night. Sleep restriction is particularly effective for those whose insomnia is secondary to chronic pain because pain sufferers generally spend large amounts of time in bed resting, napping, or simply trying to find a comfortable body position.

Changing Your Beliefs and Attitudes about Sleep

As you implement these behavioral changes in your new lifestyle, it is critical that you also examine your beliefs and attitudes about sleep and insomnia. Self-imposed pressure to achieve certain sleep standards, excessive concerns about the consequences of poor sleep, and false assumptions about sleep can feed into your sleeping problem. If you can change your unrealistic expectations regarding sleep requirements, challenge dysfunctional beliefs about the consequences of sleeplessness, and correct misattributions about the causes of insomnia, you will move a long way toward a better night's sleep.

Expectations such as "I must sleep eight hours every night" or "I must fall asleep in minutes" are unrealistic. Sleep needs vary widely among individuals and short sleep is not necessarily pathological. There is no universal standard for sleep duration. Sleep as much as you need to feel rested in the morning and remain alert during the day, but not more. Do not place pressure on yourself to achieve certain sleep standards as this will only increase your anxiety and perpetuate your insomnia. Try not to compare your sleep pattern with your bedmate's. There will always be someone who is taller, wealthier, or sleeps better than you. It is best simply to acknowledge that your bed partner falls asleep faster or sleeps longer than you do.

Attributions of insomnia to external causes are self-defeating. When you say "my sleep problem is entirely due to pain," then you assume nothing can be done about improving your sleep unless the pain is removed. By now you have learned that behavioral factors can also exacerbate sleep disturbances even though pain is a significant contributing factor. Thus it is important that you adopt a more constructive approach to beating insomnia.

Excessive worrying about the daytime consequences of a poor night's sleep only aggravates your problem. When you worry about those presumed consequences, it only makes you more anxious and decreases your tolerance for pain. You also feed into the vicious cycle of insomnia, emotional distress, low pain tolerance, and more disturbed sleep (see figure 1).

Blaming sleep for mood swings, lowered energy, increased pain, and poor daytime performance is counterproductive. There are numerous factors including natural circadian changes, hormonal changes, aging, as well as stress in other areas of your life that may cause those problems. So don't blame it all on lack of sleep.

Turning a sleepless night into a catastrophe only makes matters worse. Sleep lost is more likely to be distressing if you perceive it as stressful rather than as a challenge. Don't panic after a sleepless night; stay calm and accept the fact you didn't sleep well the night before. The only certain consequence of sleeplessness is that it will eventually lead to sleepiness. Furthermore, the positive coping strategies in chapter 6 can help you identify your self-defeating thoughts and turn them into ideas more compatible with managing pain and finding sleep.

Coping with Nocturnal Pain

A person in pain faces unique obstacles to a good night's sleep. The immediate prominence of pain is often hard to ignore and many people who suffer from chronic pain report that their pain is the main reason they have difficulty sleeping at night. There is no question that feeling pain makes it harder to relax and let go. Still, it may be inaccurate to say that the pain is entirely responsible for the insomnia. For example, when a person naps during the day and consequently is not very tired at night, it is not the pain alone that is keeping the person awake, but rather the person's poor sleep habits. Thus it is extremely important to implement all the sleep management techniques just described above. Techniques specific for coping with nocturnal pain will not be very useful if implemented separate from a total self-management program.

Relaxation

A variety of relaxation procedures are described in chapter 3; these techniques can be particularly useful for pain patients having a hard time falling or staying sleep. These exercises have proved useful in the treatment of a variety of disorders including chronic pain. Overly tense muscles are often to blame in a number of pain conditions including low-back pain, temporomandibular disorders, and headaches. Relaxation exercises produce lower levels of muscle tension and consequently lead to decreased pain levels. Many chronic pain sufferers are not aware of high levels of tension in their muscles until their muscles start to hurt. Tense muscles are a signal from your body telling you to relax. Unfortunately, most people learn to tune this message out and become quite unaware of what their bodies are trying tell them. If you practice PMR daily, you'll become more aware of high levels of tension in your muscles and be able to relax these muscles *before* they become painful. Lower levels of pain will lead to less disruption of sleep at night. By becoming proficient at the relaxation exercises, you can then derive a double benefit: you'll have more control over daytime pain, and you'll be better able to relax yourself as a sleep induction technique at night.

You may find relaxation training beneficial for its other effects as well. It has proved to be one of the most generally beneficial techniques in the whole array of psychological methods. Sometimes relaxation exercises are described as psychology's equivalent to aspirin. Learning relaxation techniques gives you a degree of mastery over your body, and this sense of control alone has beneficial effects on your sense of well-being. PMR, as outlined in chapter 3, is a good basic technique for determining your levels of muscle tension and release. A note of caution for pain patients using PMR: do not tense muscles to the point of pain. Begin these exercises slowly and progress through them gradually.

Imagery

Despite careful adherence to all of the procedures outlined here, there may be some nights when pain intensity interferes with sleep.

Fortunately, imagery is an extremely useful pain control technique that can be used in conjunction with relaxation exercises to help induce sleep. Imagery is useful in this context because it diverts your attention from something unpleasant (pain) to a more pleasant image (pain melting like ice). Numerous studies have demonstrated that when people focus their attention on their pain, they report much higher levels of pain intensity and unpleasantness than when they are distracted with another task. In the daytime it is relatively easy to distract yourself or to "take your mind off" the pain. It can be much more difficult to do so at night when there is nothing to do except try to fall asleep. At night, when the lights are off and it gets fairly quiet, the only stimuli to attend to are those created inside your own body. Unless you direct your attention away with images you create in your mind, the stimuli your body creates may be painful and hard to ignore. To create more positive mental images try following the four steps below:

1. Relax deeply (see chapter 6).
   Practice your relaxation exercises daily so that you can readily become relaxed when you need to.
2. Imagine your pain.
   Once you are proficient at the relaxation exercises, think of an image that represents the particular type, quality, and intensity of your pain.

   Some examples are pins and needles sticking in the flesh at the site of pain; a searing sun at the point of pain; a hammer pounding, or a vice turning at the site of pain.

   What's important here is for you to make the image of your pain personally meaningful.
3. Imagine your pain relief.
   Change the image of pain to something pleasant, or at least tolerable. Visualize a therapeutic image or process that represents the release of pain.

Examples of how the pain images presented in number two might be transformed could be snowflakes lying lightly on the skin that melt away instead of pins and needles in the flesh; a cooling moon replacing the sun with a gentle, soothing reflection of light; a hammer fading or dissolving away; the vice slowly opening and becoming caring, massaging hands.

Remember, conjure up these images while you are in a relaxed state. You do not have to force the images to appear; when you are relaxed, images will come to you. Select the images that are personally meaningful to you and that best depict your pain and its release.

4. Imagine the positive benefits.
Visualize yourself feeling better, smiling and laughing, moving around freely, enjoying the people and the things around you. Create an image of yourself that is active, positive, and in good health.

Many advocates of imagery training suggest that this type of imagery facilitates communication between mind and body and enhances the healing process. Although the effects of imagery on the healing process are uncertain, they are clearly not detrimental. In fact, they seem particularly helpful for coping with nocturnal pain.

Benefiting from Social Support: Family, Friends, and Work

Chronic pain sufferers are keenly aware that family and friends often fail to provide the type of social support they need or want. This is partly because the debilitating effects of chronic insomnia and chronic pain can be very difficult for others to understand if they have not experienced these problems personally. Unlike an obvious wound or a symptom that others can observe, chronic pain and insomnia are largely internal, subjective experiences. The person suffering from these symptoms generally must tell others for them to notice there is something wrong. Also, chronic pain patients have to make requests and turn down requests because of their symptoms. How these types of interactions (e.g., reporting symptoms, making or turning down requests) are approached is crucial in learning to cope with chronic pain and insomnia. Other people may want to be supportive but may not know what is needed. Consequently, they may offer too much help, or not enough, simply out of ignorance.

Research has shown that insomniacs tend to internalize their emotions and are more introverted than good sleepers. They often spend excessive amounts of time thinking about their problems, which can lead to feelings of frustration, anger, depression, or anxiety. Insomnia sufferers do not always express these emotions or communicate their needs effectively. Anger is often withheld or expressed inappropriately through a passive or an aggressive style. It is difficult then to go to bed with lingering feelings of anger or frustration and still have a good night's sleep. By dealing assertively with other people, you'll be better able to obtain the type of support you need, improve the quality of your relationship with others, and get yourself a good night's sleep.

There are essentially three different styles of relating to others: *passively, aggressively,* and *assertively.* Being assertive means expressing your thoughts, feelings, and needs while respecting those of others. Being passive and/or aggressive makes it difficult for you to communicate effectively with others and can impede your ability to have your needs met.

Passive Style

People who act in a passive or unassertive style are reluctant to express their needs to others. Passive people are usually nonresponders; when they do ask for something, it is usually in an indirect way. The needs of others are consistently placed above the needs of the self. People often adopt a passive style because they are afraid of being rejected. Often they have internalized a belief that they must be perfect, that in order to win the approval of others they must be agreeable and unimposing. For example, Jane is afraid to ask her husband to change his night owl behaviors because he works so hard, even though she has to rise at 5 A.M. to catch a train.

A passive style may lead to several problems. Resentment and anger are an almost inevitable consequence of not making your needs known. These negative emotional states can eat away at your peace of mind and diminish the quality of day-to-day living. Anger at not having your own needs met may manifest itself in more disturbed sleep and increased muscle tension and pain. Moreover, being reluctant to make or turn down requests can land you in situations that aggravate your pain or sleep problem. People don't extend invitations or make requests to make your life difficult; they just express their own needs and desires, and assume you'll do the same. Remember, there is nothing imposing about making a request or expressing a need as long as it respects the other person's right to refuse. Finally, most people find it frustrating to interact with a person behaving unassertively. It puts an unfair burden on others to read the mind or guess the needs of the person who does not express theirs. The most satisfying relationships are those in which participants feel an equal balance between having their own needs met and meeting the needs of others.

Aggressive Style

People who adopt an aggressive style, the opposite extreme, demand that their needs be met, even at the expense of others. They act as if their thoughts, feelings, and needs are the only ones that matter. People who consistently act in an aggressive manner are often fundamentally insecure people. They seem to have internalized the belief that "I must be right" to compensate for feelings of inadequacy. Challenges to that belief are threatening to their self-esteem. For example, Fred faults Jane for needing so much sleep and blames her for curtailing his fun.

There are other problems with the aggressive style. For instance, people who do not respect the thoughts and feelings and rights of others will alienate others and put them on the defensive. The frustration that often accompanies chronic pain and insomnia may foster an aggressive style. If this describes you, consider the assertive style as a more productive alternative. The aggressive style may hinder the quality of care received because it often leads to unsatisfactory relationships with health-care professionals and fosters a doctor shopping strategy. There is a difference between healthy questioning and outright challenging hostility.

Assertive Style

People with an assertive style believe that they have a legitimate right to express their own thoughts, feelings, and needs while still respecting those of others. People who adopt an assertive style have learned to express their needs directly through words and actions. They are able to listen attentively and truly "hear" the feeling and opinions of others. They can deal with criticism without becoming hostile or defensive. For example, Fred and Jane agree to problem solve an equitable solution. An assertive style can yield several benefits. Direct communication of feelings and needs fosters supportive relationships at home and at work. Moreover, assertive communication improves quality of services from health-care providers. People who ask questions and directly express their feelings and needs regarding their medical treatment set the stage for effective dialogue regarding patient care.

The following vignette describes Jack, a chronic pain patient with insomnia. The vignette is followed by several responses Jack might make. Note the differences in how Jack might respond to his problem.

Jack has suffered from chronic low-back pain for almost five years and has had chronic insomnia for almost as long. He has always thought that it was the pain that prevented him from being able to sleep at night but now realizes that there are several other factors that contribute to his poor sleep. He would like to quit using his bed as the "center of his universe," which would include no longer watching late-night TV in bed with his wife.

Response 1:

Jack gives the TV to his son Mike without telling his wife about his plans. When she acts hurt about his apparent unwillingness to watch TV with her at night Jack says "Look, I'm the one who is in pain, but you're the one who is always complaining about something. I read it right here in this book, no more watching TV in bed. If I can't watch TV in bed I don't want you doing it either. Now that's that—case closed—no more discussion." This is an example of an aggressive style.

Response 2:

Jack makes a number of changes to diminish the extent to which his bed is the center of his universe. For example, he quits writing letters and stops talking on the telephone in bed. However, Jack is reluctant to say anything to his wife about the TV since she seems to enjoy watching the late-night shows with him in bed at night. He is afraid that if he mentions anything to his wife about changing their habits she will be angry and not want to do anything with him in the evening. Jack decides that he has made enough changes and so says nothing to his wife and his old habit continues. This is an example of a passive style.

Response 3:

Jack would like to implement all the changes he has read about. He realizes that these changes will have a substantial impact on his wife's sleep habits and so he plans a time when it would be convenient to have an open discussion about proposed changes. He says to her at dinner, "I have been reading a book that makes some suggestions I think might help me sleep better at night. I would like to talk to you about it after dinner if that's okay with you." After dinner the two of them sit down together and Jack says, "I would like to try these changes to see if they help me sleep better at night. I want to know what you think about them because I know these changes will affect you as well." Jack and his wife decide to watch TV in the living room together before retiring for the evening. This is an example of an assertive style.

Social Support Groups

Though relationships at home and work will be more satisfying if you adopt an assertive style, you may still feel a need to interact with people who are experiencing the same types of problems as yourself. Support groups bring together people who share similar experiences, allowing them to empathize with one another and share coping strategies. A support group can provide a safe environment in which to practice new interpersonal skills, receive feedback and advice regarding coping strategies, and hear fresh perspectives on familiar difficulties. Social support groups are usually not places where people commiserate with a "life's a bitch and then you die" philosophy. A support group provides sympathy for problems from a first-person perspective, but it also encourages people to cope adaptively with their limitations, and take a positive, proactive stance toward their problems. Social support has proved a very helpful supplement to this self-management program in the treatment of chronic pain and insomnia.

Summary

Chronic pain complicates your insomnia problem, as sleep disturbances complicate your experience with pain and illness. But there is a way to regain control and break this cycle. This self-management program is a highly structured regimen that requires time, patience, and commitment if you expect sleep to improve. Psychological research has shown that successful management of insomnia associated with chronic pain requires consistent adherence to this regimen for eight to ten weeks. The self-management approach implies that you take responsibility for implementing the recommended changes and that you take an active role in the treatment process. Diligent adherence to the clinical procedures is often the key to a successful outcome. You may find that your sleep pattern gets worse the first few nights of practice and that you wake up in the morning feeling more exhausted than usual. Do not get discouraged. With time and repeated practice, your sleep pattern will improve. If you faithfully implement the techniques described in this chapter but continue to experience insomnia secondary to chronic pain, it is a good idea to consult your physician regarding referral to a sleep clinic or a multidisciplinary pain clinic. You can benefit from the additional support and reinforcement of other patients, as well as careful guidance from health-care professionals in correcting any errors or resistance interfering with the process of regaining control of your sleep.

Sleep Disorders

12

Most poor sleepers can learn to manage insomnia through behavioral techniques such as proper sleep hygiene and relaxation. But some forms of insomnia have underlying physical disorders that may require careful medical attention. These disorders can be mere annoyances, as with teeth grinding (bruxism), or potentially life threatening, as with sleep apnea.

The Epworth Sleepiness Scale

The Epworth Sleepiness Scale (ESS) was developed and validated by Dr. Murray Johns of Melbourne, Australia. It is a simple, self-administered questionnaire that is widely used by sleep professionals in quantifying the level of daytime sleepiness.

How likely are you to doze off or to fall asleep in the following situations, in contrast to just feeling tired? This refers to your usual way of life in recent times. Even if you have not done some of these things recently, try to work out how they would have affected you.

Use the following scale to choose the most appropriate number for each situation:

0—Would *never* doze
1—*Slight* chance of dozing
2—*Moderate* chance of dozing
3—*High* chance of dozing

Situation	Chance of Dozing
Sitting and reading	_____
Watching TV	_____
Sitting inactive in a public place (e.g., a theater or meeting)	_____
As a passenger in a car for an hour without a break	_____
Lying down to rest in the afternoon when circumstances permit	_____
Sitting and talking to someone	_____
Sitting quietly after lunch without alcohol	_____
In a car while stopped for a few minutes in traffic	_____
Total Score:	_____

Scoring Key:
1–6: Congratulations, you are getting enough sleep.
7–8: Your score is average.
9 and up: Seek the advice of a sleep specialist without delay.

Sources: Johns, M.W. "A new method for measuring daytime sleepiness: the Epworth Sleepiness Scale." *Sleep* 1991; 14: 540–5, and Dr. William Dement at the Stanford University Web site.

Before you decide that you definitely do or do not suffer from one of the disorders described in this chapter, it can be a good idea to have yourself evaluated at a qualified sleep center. You can find a sleep center near you by checking out one of the Web sites/addresses listed at the end of this book. Sleep apnea and narcolepsy are serious enough to require professional consultation; sleep specialists will be able to provide you with appropriate diagnosis, treatment, and medication. This chapter is intended to give you a brief but comprehensive overview of the most common physical disorders affecting sleep quality. For a thorough description of what you might experience in a sleep center, please refer to chapter 11.

The most life threatening sleep disorder is sleep apnea, sometimes called the "snoring sickness." This is the most common of all physically based sleep disorders, and is discussed first. The following sections cover PLM and RLS, which inhibit sleep onset. Both of these disorders occur in only a small percentage of the adult population. Next is narcolepsy, or excessive daytime sleepiness. This is the least common of all sleep disorders, but it can be extremely disruptive to your life.

Finally, RBD is not quite considered a parasomnia (described below), but is being studied for organic causes.

Another category of disorder is termed "parasomnias," or disorders of partial arousal. While the disorders previously mentioned are believed to have a strong organic (physical) component, the parasomnias are more behaviorally based and occur for the most part in childhood. A small percentage of the adult population does experience parasomnias, however. The most commonly acknowledged parasomnias are sleep walking (or somnabulism), night terrors, nightmares, teeth grinding (or bruxism). The other most commonly recognized parasomnia is nocturnal enuresis, or bedwetting, which is not covered in this book. For further discussion of parasomnias, please refer to chapter 8.

While sleep apnea, narcolepsy, and restless legs have little in common symptomatically, they do share two similarities: they have an underlying physical cause, and they significantly reduce your sleep and life quality. Don't hesitate to seek adequate professional help for these troublesome disorders.

Sleep Apnea—The Snoring Sickness

It has long been a myth that loud snoring signifies a sound sleeper. Snoring, however, is now known to signal a potentially life threatening disorder: sleep apnea. As Dr. Dement writes, "In a stunning evolutionary failure, nature endowed us with throats that tend to collapse during sleep and stop air flow, but did not endow our sleeping brains with the ability to start breathing again calmly."

Most people suffering from sleep apnea are unaware of its disruptive symptoms throughout the night. They wake up feeling unrefreshed and struggle through the day in a fatigued state, yet are unaware that they probably woke up hundreds of times throughout the night gasping for air. Often it is the bedmate who alerts sleep experts of the loud choking, gasping, and nonstop snoring sounds of the sleep apnea sufferer.

Sleep apnea sufferers generally breathe normally during the day, but their breathing becomes shallow at night. At times it ceases altogether for a few seconds and for up to two minutes. This can cause partial or complete arousal from sleep and may go on all night. Males seem to develop this condition more often than females, and there is evidence that it appears more frequently in the elderly. Other factors that may play a part in contributing to sleep apnea are obesity and short, thick necks. Those who have narcolepsy tend to develop sleep apnea more often than the population as a whole. The only way to make a definite diagnosis of this condition is to be evaluated overnight in a sleep lab.

Experts describe three types of sleep apnea:

Central Apnea is relatively rare and found in those whose chief complaints are insomnia and excessive sleepiness. Central apnea is thought to originate in the brain, which sends a message to the diaphragm to stop moving in and out with air intake and exhalation, causing breathing to stop altogether. The sleeper must wake up several times a night to resume breathing.

Obstructive Apnea, also known as "upper airway sleep apnea," is more common than central sleep apnea. In this condition, the diaphragm is not involved. Muscles of the upper airway (tongue, throat, and pharynx) relax so significantly that the throat collapses and breathing is completely blocked. The sleeper usually does not remember gasping for air many times a night, and loudly snoring.

Mixed Sleep Apnea is a combination of the above two conditions and consists of a brief period of central apnea followed by a longer period of obstructive apnea.

The American Sleep Apnea Association lists the following facts about sleep apnea on its Web site:

- Sleep apnea is very common, as common as adult diabetes, and affects more than twelve million Americans.
- Risk factors include being male, overweight, and over the age of forty.
- However, it can strike anyone at any age, including children.
- Untreated, sleep apnea can cause high blood pressure and other cardiovascular disease, memory problems, weight gain, impotency, and headaches.
- Untreated sleep apnea may be responsible for job impairment and motor vehicle crashes.

Treatment

The most frequently and successfully used method of treatment for sleep apnea is CPAP (Continuous Positive Airway Pressure). This mechanical device can be rented from home health-care companies and consists of a portable generator, a tube, and a mask. The device gently blows air into your mouth and nose to prevent collapse of the upper airway muscles and eliminate snoring. It makes only a light noise that is not disruptive to you or your bedmate.

Doctors can prescribe certain medications such as protripty-line and progesterone to stimulate breathing. In addition, they will encourage the sleep apnea sufferer to lose weight, stop smoking (which irritates the upper airway), avoid alcohol, use a vaporizer to keep airways clear of congestion, and use pillows to elevate the head. Some devices are recommended, such as mouth guards, for obstructive sleep apnea. Simple corrective surgery may also be recommended, where the interior of the throat is enlarged. Or, for severe cases of sleep apnea—one hundred or more interruptions in breathing in six hours of sleep—a tracheostomy is performed. This relatively simple surgery involves inserting a tube into the windpipe, bypassing the throat area and allowing air to pass directly into the lungs. The tube is removed during the day to allow for a normal social life.

A word of caution: unless carefully monitored and administered, drugs can be fatal to a sleep apnea sufferer. This condition puts a severe strain on the cardiac system due to constant awakenings. In addition, the sedating effects of alcohol, tranquilizers, and sleeping pills can further aggravate and depress the respiratory system. Be sure to check with your health-care professional and/or a sleep lab expert to determine the appropriate kind and amount of medication.

Periodic Limb Movement Disorder (PLM)

Formally known as nocturnal myoclonus, sufferers of PLM experience nightly muscle movements, sometimes very violent and usually in the legs. Typically they are not aware of these intermittent and rhythmic leg jerks and must rely on a bed partner to clue them in to their kicking and fitful sleep. Some people who have this unusual disorder are partially or completely awakened in the night and report fatigue and lethargy the next day. This disorder runs in families, becomes more frequent and severe with age, and must be confirmed by an evaluation in a sleep lab.

Treatment

The cause of PLM is unknown. Treatment consists of regular exercise and a drug called clonazepam.

Restless Legs Syndrome (RLS)

Sometimes known as "nervous legs," this disorder is similar to PLM in that its origin is unknown and sufferers experience leg jerks. However, it occurs mostly as the person is trying to fall asleep, making it difficult for him to relax enough to go to sleep. One patient describes this disorder as "uncomfortable but not painful sensations creeping deep inside the calf." Studies show that RLS becomes more severe with age, sleep deprivation, and pregnancy.

Treatment

Moving about often relieves the discomfort. Also, an adequate exercise program combined with some form of muscle relaxation has brought relief to some people with this disorder. RLS runs in families and may be due to poor circulation. Medications such as carbidopa and levodopa (also used for Parkinson's disease) have also been proven effective. Most people with restless leg syndrome also have Periodic Limb Movement Disorder.

Narcolepsy

People with narcolepsy are sometimes regarded as "lazy" and "incompetent" because they will suddenly and without apparent reason fall soundly asleep in the middle of daily activities such as eating, talking, even driving. These sleep attacks can last anywhere from a few seconds to more than thirty minutes. Narcoleptics may not even be aware that they suffer from this devastating disease, only that they regularly experience chronic fatigue. Sometimes these minisleeps can be a mere annoyance, but they can be disastrous when they cause accidents or trouble holding down a job. The Stanford School of Medicine reports in its current Web site that narcolepsy is a very disabling and underdiagnosed illness. It is the second leading cause of excessive daytime sleepiness diagnosed by sleep centers after obstructive sleep apnea. Dr. Dement of Stanford University reported in 1983 that in an AMA study of narcoleptics, 41 percent had occupational disabilities, 89 percent had deteriorating relationships, and 91 percent had accidents they attributed to their sleepiness. The exact physical mechanism causing narcolepsy is unknown, although it is thought to be a defect in central nervous system functioning.

Usually there is a family history of narcolepsy, with males and females equally affected. The first signs routinely appear in the early teens and twenties, and symptoms worsen with age.

Another sign of narcolepsy is excessive daytime sleepiness (EDS), also often referred to as "sleep attacks." These attacks usually last ten to fifteen minutes, unless the person is lying or sitting, in which case sleep may last two to three hours.

Narcoleptics often awake fully refreshed from these sleep attacks. However, their regular nighttime sleep is usually disturbed by multiple awakenings, temporary suspension of breathing (similar to sleep apnea—see the previous section), restlessness, nightmares, and disturbing images upon sleep onset and awakening, called hypnagogic hallucinations. Narcoleptics rarely feel fully alert and refreshed through the day, even after extended sleep.

About 60 percent of all narcoleptics experience cataplexy, a brief or sudden loss of muscle control. This muscle weakness can last several minutes and result in a physical collapse; the person experiences paralysis but remains fully or partially conscious. These attacks are usually triggered by emotions such as laughter, excitement, and anger. For this reason, some narcoleptics try not to respond emotionally and may in fact avoid situations likely to evoke strong emotions.

Narcoleptics typically fall asleep in less than five minutes (compared to an average of twelve to twenty minutes for most adults to fall asleep) and go immediately into REM sleep, the stage where most dreaming occurs. The normal adult population moves into REM in about ninety minutes. This immediate intrusion of REM into the narcoleptic's sleep may account for the sometimes terrifying hypnagogic hallucinations, which occur right at the beginning and end of sleep. These hallucinations are vivid, dreamlike images that are not uncommon among most people. However, narcoleptics experience them immediately upon falling asleep, during a cataplectic episode, and sometimes when fully conscious.

Sleep paralysis is sometimes a symptom of narcolepsy, where sufferers feel as if they cannot move a single muscle when falling asleep or waking up. This feeling can last for a few seconds or up to several minutes. Sleep paralysis combined with hypnagogic hallucinations are less frequent than the first two symptoms (EDS and cataplexy) but are terrifying nonetheless.

Harvey, an office worker, has had bouts of sleep paralysis since childhood. He remains fully conscious, but can't move a single muscle, except a finger. He has learned to wiggle that finger until he wakes up. "If I roll over right away and don't get up," he says, "I'll fall right back into that paralyzed state." Harvey, whose roots are in the southeastern United States, has elderly relatives who call this condition having a "hag riding your back." Evidently the imaginary hag, or witch, needs to harass the sleeper. Southern folklore has it that if you leave a broom by your bed, the witch will be preoccupied counting the bristles and won't ride your back!

13

Medications for Sleep

As you have read in the previous chapters, knowledge of the types of insomnia and the variety of possible causes has increased greatly during the past three decades. This knowledge has affected the way sleeping medications are used in medical practice. More specific treatments are becoming available for some types of insomnia; more is known about the classes of drugs commonly prescribed. Most experts believe that pharmacological treatment for sleep disturbance can be helpful for certain patients when an appropriate evaluation has been undertaken. They also agree on some common caveats and precautions. This chapter will focus on the advantages and disadvantages of medications commonly used to promote sleep. Your doctor can help you determine what medications—if any—are best for you. Educating yourself, as well, as to the options available, will help you participate in the decision and weigh the risks and benefits.

To quote a legend in the field, Dr. Dement in *The Promise of Sleep* puts sleep medications in perspective. "Sleeping pills are haunted by an inglorious past, even though today's medications are far safer and more sophisticated. . . . The history of drug development for insomnia has been a quest to develop sleep-inducing medications that are safe at higher doses, are not addictive, wear off quickly so that the user doesn't feel sleepy the next day, and don't have side effects."

Several different types of drugs are prescribed to improve sleep; others are used for this purpose even though they may be prescribed for other reasons. The most commonly prescribed drugs are the BZDs, also known as anxiolytics, which relieve anxiety, a common reason for insomnia. Other prescription drugs include barbiturates and antidepressants. Nonprescription, or OTC, drugs are often self-administered to combat sleep difficulty, as is alcohol. In some instances illegal drugs such as marijuana are used for sleep induction. In one sense, then, all of these can be considered "sleeping pills" or "sleeping medications." As you might guess, some are far less advisable than others.

All prescription sleeping medications alter the sleep stages that occur as you sleep. In general, these drugs decrease stage one—light, transitional sleep—while increasing stage two. At higher doses, REM sleep slow-wave sleep may also be suppressed. Although decreasing light sleep seems desirable, the significance of decreasing SWS or REM sleep is not fully understood. Some experts believe that slow wave sleep represents the "best" or "deepest," most restorative sleep. If REM is significantly suppressed by a drug, abrupt discontinuation of the drug typically leads to an increase in REM sleep. This "REM rebound" may be associated with vivid dreaming, possibly even nightmares. This same phenomenon occurs if REM is suppressed without medication. It suggests that REM sleep must be made up if lost. Nevertheless, no behavioral consequences have been noted even when REM is markedly reduced for weeks or months. REM rebound is not physically dangerous, but keep in mind that in some cases unpleasant, vivid dreams may occur.

Side Effects and Daytime Functioning

Most sleeping medications fall into the class of drugs known as sedative-hypnotics. Hypnotic medications reduce alertness and promote sleepiness. In cases of insomnia, this is usually a desired effect. However, this sedation can become a side effect (an undesired effect) with the passage of time. One type of side effect occurs when the sedating properties of a sleeping pill given at night continue into the waking hours. This can cause individuals to feel even worse during the daytime than they commonly feel following a night of disturbed sleep. More important, alertness and performance may be significantly impaired. The goal of treatment is to improve daytime functioning as well as sleep. Thus a sleeping medication that improves sleep significantly but results in daytime sleepiness or "morning hangover" has not met this goal. A sleeping pill with a long duration of action is much more likely to produce carry-over effects than one with a shorter duration of action, because the long-acting medication stays in the body for a longer period of time than the short-acting medication. Also, the higher the dose, the longer the medication may remain pharmacologically active, and the greater the likelihood of interfering with daytime functioning.

Tolerance

Chronic use of sedative-hypnotics can in some cases lead to the development of tolerance to the medication. This means a previously effective amount of medication becomes ineffective over time, usually a period of weeks or months. As tolerance develops, the sleep disturbance returns, and may encourage the user to increase the dosage of medication. If this pattern is repeated often enough, it may result in drug dependency along with persistent sleep disturbance. Therefore, it is usually wise to limit nightly use of sleep medications to short periods of time, or to use them a few nights per week. The dose of the drug should not be increased, once an effective dose has been established.

Discontinuation Effects

Sleeping pills rarely "cure" the insomnia. That is, they do not very often, if ever, correct whatever factors are leading to the insomnia. It should not be surprising, then, to learn that if the medication is stopped, the sleep disturbance returns. In some cases, discontinuation of sedative-hypnotic medication, particularly after high doses, may result in a few nights of sleep disturbances that is more severe than was present before treatment. This withdrawal effect often includes REM rebound, and is termed "rebound insomnia." If the withdrawal effects are particularly severe, you may be tempted to return to use of the medication. Avoiding dosages greater than the lowest effective dose will minimize the likelihood of rebound insomnia.

The BZDs are now the most commonly prescribed medication to promote sleep. In the United States, there are three benzodiazepines that currently have FDA approval for treatment of insomnia: flurazepam (Dalmane), temazepan (Restoril), and triazolam (Halcion). A number of others are marketed as antianxiety agents but are also used as sleeping pills (see table on page 182). There are several non–BZD compounds available for insomnia as well. Research studies have consistently demonstrated that BZDs reduce the time it takes for people to fall asleep, reduce the number and length of awakenings at night, and, as a result, increase total sleep time. Other types of medications (e.g., barbiturates) have a smaller margin between effective dose and the dose that produces serious reactions. Thus, overdosing on BZDs is much less likely than with other sleeping pills.

Another reason that BZDs are relatively safe medications is that they do not interact with many other medications. That is, they will not influence the effectiveness or safety of most other medications a person may be taking for other health problems (although there are exceptions). In contrast, barbiturates have a greater potential for changing the effects of other medications. This does not mean, however, that it is safe to drink alcohol or take certain prescription pain medication while taking BZDs. The sedating effects of BZDs will be intensified by alcohol and other central nervous system depressant drugs (e.g., codeine) and therefore these drugs should not be used in combination.

Even though BZDs are safer than other sleep medications, they must be approached with caution. Abrupt termination of long-term, very high-dosage BZD use has been shown to trigger serious, possibly life-threatening, symptoms such as seizures, high fever, panic reactions, hallucinations, and delusions. There have even been reports of some withdrawal symptoms after long-term use of moderate doses of BZDs, but there are no controlled studies to substantiate these reports. Because of differing sensitivities to drugs of this type, withdrawal from long-term or high-dose BZD use should always be performed under the supervision of a physician using gradual reductions in your dose so that symptoms can be minimized.

Antidepressant drugs with sedative effects are occasionally prescribed for the treatment of insomnia in patients who are not depressed. Unfortunately, little objective research has examined the effects of these drugs in nondepressed insomnia patients. However, antidepressants may have reduced the likelihood of dependence or abuse compared to BZDs. Depressed individuals who take antidepressants often experience improvement in their sleep. But the drug's primary effect is on the depression, not on the insomnia. Research has yet to determine the benefits—and drawbacks—of antidepressants for nondepressed insomniacs.

Specific Medications for Insomnia

Sleep medications, sometimes called "hypnotic medications," generally should not be the treatment of first choice for chronic insomnia. However, judicious use of hypnotics may be helpful when treating transient or short-term insomnia, but their use should be restricted to less than four weeks' duration. Intermittent use of hypnotics (one to two nights per week) may be necessary in some patients with chronic insomnia who do not respond adequately to nonpharmacologic treatment. This also means that if hypnotics are prescribed, they should always be combined with behavioral therapies such as relaxation training, diet, exercise and sleep hygiene.

Typical hypnotics

Generic Name	Trade Name
Anxiolytics:	
Diazepam	Valium
Lorazepam	Ativan
Benzodiazepines (BZDs):	
Flurazepam	Dalmane
Temazepam	Restoril
Estazolam	ProSom
Triazolam	Halcion

The elimination half-lifes (the time for the body to excrete half of the drug) of sedative-hypnotics vary widely. This is important to know, because adverse events such as memory impairments, falls, and daytime sleepiness occur at longer half lives. Keep in mind that the elimination of such drugs, even the shortest acting, is slowed down in the geriatric population because of age-related impairments in renal (kidney) function and sometimes in liver function.

BZDs

Flurazepam is the longest acting, with a half-life of 36 to 120 hours. This means the drug effect lingers from at least a day and a half to five days. As stated above, the use of this medication could lead to daytime sleepiness, cognitive impairment, lack of coordination, and worsening of any preexisting depression.

Temazepam and estazolam have intermediate elimination half-lifes of ten to twenty-four hours and consequently are less likely to be associated with daytime sleepiness.

Triazolam binds to specific sites in the brain called GABA receptors. Triazolam stimulates these receptors, making the neurons (brain cells) less excitable and more stable, producing a calming effect. Triazolam has a very short half-life of two to five hours. This means that half of the drug is gone in two to five hours, which means that some is still present after six to seven hours. Triazolam can cause anterograde amnesia, which is the inability to retain new information. Similar to all other benzodiazepines, it has been associated with dependence and withdrawal. Decreasing the dose or stopping the medication can cause some adverse events, including seizures.

A Note about BZDs

BZDs should be avoided or used judiciously in alcoholics or patients who have kidney, liver, or lung disease. This class of drugs should also be avoided in patients who have sleep apnea.

Nonbenzodiazepines

Zolpidem is structurally different from benzodiazepines and exerts its effect on the same GABA receptors as triazolam. It retains most if not all of the BZD hypnotic and much of the anxiolytic (anxiety relieving) properties. However, it is less likely than the

BZDs to disturb the architecture of sleep and to cause mental and psychiatric side effects. Its onset of action is within thirty minutes and its duration is six to eight hours. It has the same adverse side effects as BZDs, such as being habit forming. Elderly and debilitated patients taking this medication should be monitored closely for impaired cognitive or motor performance.

Zaleplon (Sonata) is not related to BZDs, however, it interacts with the same GABA receptor complex. Onset of its effect is within one hour; its duration is six to eight hours. The spectrum of side effects is very similar to zolpidem.

Antidepressants

Trazadone (Desyrel) increases the level of one of the brain chemicals or neurotransmitters called serotonin, a naturally occurring chemical believed to be involved in creating feelings of well-being. It decreases the sensitivity of some of the stimulant receptors, and blocks histamine receptors, which is responsible in part for its sedative properties. Although helpful and widely prescribed for many people, strictly speaking, it is not FDA approved for use in the treatment of insomnia.

In general, judicious use of hypnotics in the treatment of insomnia is recommended for all age groups. In the elderly population, preferable medications for short-term use are the short-acting BZDs, zolpidem or zalephon, but generally not for more than four weeks. Overall, hypnotics should not be the major component of therapy for insomnia. Attention to psychological and environmental issues should be the first line of treatment.

Treatment of Primary Sleep Disorders

As well as BZDs, carbidopa/levodopa (trade name Sinemet) and gabapentin (trade name Neurontin) have been used to treat PLM, but they are not official FDA-approved uses.

Restless Legs Syndrome has been successfully treated with carbamazepine (trade name Tegretol), gabapentin (Neurontin), and anti-Parkinson's medications. Again, these treatments are "off label," meaning they can be commonly prescribed by physicians but are not officially indicated for that use by the FDA.

RBD has two current treatments available: clonazepam (85 percent to 90 percent effective) and melatonin, 3–9 mg (85 percent to 100 percent effective). Use of clonazepan is again not officially approved for this use by the FDA.

Over-the-Counter (OTC) Medications

Medications marketed as sleep aids are available without a doctor's prescription and are known by such familiar names as Nytol and Sominex. Most of these compounds contain an antihistamine as the sedating agent, as well as other ingredients. In many individuals, antihistamines can produce drowsiness, encouraging you to fall asleep. However, you face the same problem as with some prescription medications—they lose effectiveness over time. In addition, you may experience grogginess and lack of focus the next day. Given the little evidence that insomnia over the long run is significantly improved with such OTC medications, you would be wise to speak with your health-care practitioner before relying solely on these medications for sleep.

Benadryl: (The "PM" of Tylenol PM and Sominex are examples of OTC medications)

Benadryl primarily blocks histamine receptors, giving you relief from colds and allergies. However, it was also noted to have a sedative effect. Now a popular OTC medication for insomnia, this drug has a half-life of 8.5 to 10 hours in healthy adults and much longer than that in elderly patients. It can interfere with alertness, can cause daytime sedation, and prolonged reaction time on the day following use. Dizziness, dryness of the mouth, constipation, blurring of vision, and confusion can occur. It is preferable not to use this medication in older people.

Alcohol (A Variation of OTC Medication)

It is not uncommon for individuals to use alcohol as a sleep inducer. Because it is a potent central nervous system sedative, sleep onset is hastened. However, tolerance to this effect occurs fairly rapidly. What's more, though alcohol may help induce sleep, sleep in the latter portions of the night becomes disturbed. As the alcohol is metabolized, the sedative effect wears off and a marked arousal response may occur due to sympathetic nervous system activity. The result may range from shallow fragmented sleep, if alcohol consumption was moderate, to long periods of wakefulness after heavy drinking. The net effect is generally a less refreshing night of sleep. Tolerance, dependence, and discontinuation effects are also significant concerns when alcohol is used as a sleep aid. Tolerance to alcohol develops rapidly, often prompting the individual to drink a larger quantity for the desired sedating effect.

Discontinuation of alcohol leads to profoundly disturbed sleep, which is likely to persist for several weeks to many months after alcohol is completely discontinued. Experts strongly advise not using alcohol to promote sleep.

Sleep Medication: Not a Cure

So many physical, psychological, and behavioral factors are known to be causes of insomnia, it seems logical that no single medication, or class of medication, could be beneficial for all patients. Indeed, this is the case. Further, sleeping medications of any type provide only symptomatic relief. This means that although sleep may be improved, the drugs have no direct effect on the cause of the insomnia. *There is no pharmacological cure for insomnia.* Because of this, it is now recognized that treatment of persistent insomnia must focus on the underlying cause(s) of the condition rather than simply producing sleep pharmacologically. This does not mean that medication should never be used in an adjunctive fashion for chronic insomnia. That is, while the underlying causes of disrupted sleep are being addressed directly, relief might be provided *temporarily* for the patient in the form of a sleeping medication. Additionally, as noted above, medications can be useful in some cases of transient or short-term insomnia.

Transient and Short-term Insomnia

Transient insomnia refers to sleep disruption for as little as a single night or as long as a week. Most people have experienced transient insomnia at some point in their lives—when starting a new job perhaps, taking college entrance examinations, or facing any momentous or nonroutine event. Even the common cold can disturb sleep for a few days. On most nights, sleep is not a problem for these individuals, but when exciting or worrisome situations occur, sleep may be affected until the situation is resolved. Transient insomnia may also occur if you attempt to sleep "out of sync" with the twenty-four-hour sleepiness/alertness rhythm (see chapter 7 for a discussion of circadian rhythms). Part of the jet lag syndrome involves poor sleep because rapid travel across time zones results in a inability of the sleep-wake rhythm to adjust rapidly to new environmental times. Therefore, the brain may be in an alert phase when local time indicates it's time to sleep. The result is light, fragmented, and often shortened sleep.

Similarly, shift workers are required to sleep during a relatively alert portion of their sleep-wake rhythm when working the night shift (usually 11 P.M. to 7 A.M.). With night work, daytime sleep is generally shortened significantly. In most cases, people simply tolerate these occasional nights of poor sleep, especially if they feel that there is usually no major consequences the following day. However, if the sleep disturbance persists for a few days, or if you can anticipate a situation that may produce a poor night of sleep when you need to be at your best the next day, you might seek medical help. A physician can recommend a medication best suited to your transient sleep difficulties.

Short-term insomnia is a sleep disruption that lasts from one week to a few months. Like transient insomnia, it is usually "triggered" by specific events such as the death of someone close, medical illness, or other stressors. Mrs. R, a middle-aged woman who is very active in community groups, is an example of an individual with short-term insomnia. When confronted with a challenge in her group activities, Mrs. R has a hard time sleeping until she has arrived at a plan of action. On the average, Mrs. R would have two or three weeks of poor sleep about every six months when a new, interesting challenge confronted her. Mrs. R could predict when sleep would be a problem and was bothered considerably by poor sleep. During the day she felt irritable and lacked the energy to resolve her newest issue. On occasion, she would fall asleep unintentionally during meetings, which was quite embarrassing. She sought help from her physician during short-term insomnia episodes. Use of sleeping pills allowed her to tolerate the stress of her activities much better by preventing sleep loss. Of course, if short-term insomnia is rooted in external causes, it's a good idea to work on those issues directly—even if you can rest with medication. Making behavioral changes may be a way to prevent your short-term insomnia from developing into a chronic problem. The key to determining if a sleep problem is transient or short term, is knowing your history of normal sleep before the causal situation occurs and after it is removed. If you can predict periods of poor sleep, and feel that you are affected significantly the next day, you may wish to discuss intermittent use of sleeping pills with your physician.

Before considering sleep medication, make sure that you follow the sleep hygiene advice in chapter 2. Some of your habits or behaviors that generally do not result in sleep problems may contribute to the problem in times of stress. For example, a cup or two of caffeinated coffee after dinner may not typically disturb your sleep enough for you to perceive it, but when you are also anxious and worried about something, the combination of caffeine and anxiety may produce considerable sleep difficulty. Eliminate those behaviors that may be contributing to transient insomnia before considering a pharmacological treatment.

Persistent (Chronic) Insomnia

Sleep medication alone is rarely, if ever, the solution for insomnia that lasts a few months or longer. Persistent insomnia is the result of a cause or causes that will not spontaneously resolve itself, often from chronic medical or psychological disorders. In some cases, the insomnia is due to a primary sleep disorder (e.g., sleep apnea). Although in many cases sleep can be improved temporarily with a sleeping pill, the underlying cause of insomnia remains. When the medication is discontinued, the sleep disruption returns. For this reason, treatment of chronic insomnia must first focus on the *cause* of the sleep problem. A specific treatment program (behavioral, psychological, or medical) must be directed at that cause for long-term benefit. For example, a patient who has difficulty falling asleep and staying asleep related to arthritic pain would undergo appropriate treatment for arthritis, such as anti-inflammatory or analgesic medications, or physical therapy. A patient who experiences early morning awakenings secondary to depression would be treated for depression with antidepressant medication and/or psychotherapy. Usually, sleep will improve as the distressing factor is eased.

In some cases, poor sleep will continue despite treatment of the underlying condition. A physician may then choose to provide relief with sleep medication even for chronic insomnia problems. At this point it is usually advisable for sleep medication to be given only for a week or two, or if a longer period is needed, for a few days per week, rather than every night. Careful attention to sleep hygiene, and an exploration of behavioral treatment options, may avert the need for pharmacological treatment.

General Precautions

Before prescribing a sleeping medication, your physician will want to know specific details about your medical history and medication use. There are several types of patients who should not take sedative-hypnotic medication. These include patients with a history of loud snoring or breathing disorders that might be worsened with ingestion of a sedative, women who are pregnant or breast-feeding, individuals with a history of drug abuse, those taking certain medications that may interact with a sedative, and those whose occupational demands require them to be capable of functioning well upon awakening in the middle of their sleep period (e.g., firemen, physicians, caregivers). If you take sleeping medication, keep in mind that carry-over sedation may be present the following day. Avoid driving or operating dangerous machinery if you do not feel alert. Realize, too, that one or two nights of disturbed sleep may be experienced following discontinuation of medication, and that this is not sufficient reason to resume taking medication. Never increase dosage of medication without the approval of your physician. In addition, do not drink alcohol if you are taking sedative-hypnotics; the interaction of the two sedatives reduces the safety margin. Remember that drug therapy is only a temporary treatment or a supplement to a more comprehensive treatment, never a cure for sleep difficulty.

Summary

In this era of immediate gratification, it's far too easy for people to grab a "quick fix" for just about anything that ails them. They are tempted to choose fast-acting pills over such things as meditation and imagery, which require more patience and practice. They disregard the negative effects of instant gratification that can result in addiction, and in the end, increased sleeplessness. It is worth your time to practice sensible sleep hygiene and stress reduction techniques such as those outlined in this book, in lieu of a quick fix. In doing so, the quality of life you experience overall will benefit many aspects of your waking life as well as your sleep.

14

Complementary and Alternative Medicine (CAM)

A growing body of unconventional wisdom supports the use of complementary and alternative medicine to aid, manage, and heal whatever ails. The interest in and use of herbs, for example, has been around for thousands of years; aromatherapy's popularity is more recent. In part this interest stems from the expense and frustration with conventional medicine. People simply cannot afford medical care, or they distrust the care they are getting. For example, Christopher Hobbs writes in *Herbal Remedies for Dummies,* "When you have trouble getting to sleep, you can grow valerian in your backyard, dig the aromatic roots, wash them, brew them and drink a strong cup of tea before bedtime—all at a minimal cost, with no prescription or examination required."

There are CAM caveats, however, just as there are with conventional medicine. Plus, there are so many opinions available about this herb or that, which exercise to use, homeopathy versus Chinese medicine, that it is easy to get confused. Before abruptly casting off your traditional doctor's opinion and wandering down an ineffective path, you would be wise to have a conversation with your health-care provider about CAM. Consult some of the excellent references available to you in books and on the internet. Talk to a trained herbalist or naturopath. Gather as much information as you can about your particular situation, knowing that one size does not fit all. You will likely need to experiment with and customize a program to fit your unique insomnia needs.

The National Institutes of Health support the NCCAM, whose Web site provides the following definition of CAM:

> A group of diverse medical and health care systems, practices and products that are not presently considered to be part of conventional medicine. While some scientific evidence exists regarding some CAM therapies, for most there are key questions that are yet to be answered through well-designed scientific studies—questions such as whether they are safe and whether they work for the diseases or medical conditions for which they are used. The list of what is considered to be CAM changes continually, as those therapies that are proven to be safe and effective become adopted into conventional health care and as new approaches to health care emerge.

It may be helpful to you to know the definitions of the various terms and practitioners of CAM as you seek out experts for support. The NCCAM Web site provides us with this handy dictionary of terms:

Aromatherapy: Aromatherapy involves the use of essential oils (extracts or essences) from flowers, herbs, and trees to promote health and well-being.

Chiropractic: Chiropractic focuses on the relationship between bodily structure (primarily that of the spine) and function, and how that relationship affects the preservation and restoration of health. Chiropractors use manipulative therapy as an integral treatment tool.

Dietary supplements: Congress defined the "dietary supplement" in the Dietary Supplement Health and Education Act (DSHEA) of 1994 as a product (other than tobacco) taken by mouth that contains a "dietary ingredient" intended to supplement the diet. Dietary ingredients may include vitamins, minerals, herbs, or other botanicals, amino acids, and substances such as enzymes, organ tissues, and metabolites. Dietary supplements come in many forms, including extracts, concentrates, tablets, capsules, gelcaps, liquids, and powders. They have special requirements for labeling. Under DSHEA, dietary supplements are considered foods, not drugs.

Electromagnetic fields: Electromagnetic fields (EMFs, also called electric and magnetic fields) are invisible lines of force that surround all electrical devices. The earth also produces EMFs; electric fields are produced when there is thunderstorm activity, and magnetic fields are believed to be produced by electric currents flowing at the earth's core.

Homeopathic medicine: In homeopathic medicine, there is a belief that "like cures like" meaning that small, highly diluted quantities of medicinal substances are given to cure symptoms, when the same substances given at higher or more concentrated doses would actually cause those symptoms.

Massage: Massage therapists manipulate muscle and connective tissue to enhance function of those tissues and promote relaxation and well-being.

Naturopathic medicine: Naturopathic practitioners work with natural healing forces within the body, with a goal of helping the body heal from disease and attain better health. Practices may include dietary modifications, massage, exercise, acupuncture, minor surgery, and various other interventions.

Osteopathic medicine: Osteopathic medicine is a form of conventional medicine that, in part, emphasizes diseases arising in the musculoskeletal system. There is an underlying belief that all of the body's systems work together, and disturbances in one system may affect function elsewhere in the body. Some osteopathic physicians practice osteopathic manipulation, a full-body system of hands-on techniques to alleviate pain, restore function, and promote health and well-being.

Qi gong: Qi gong is a component of traditional Chinese medicine that combines movement, meditation, and regulation of breathing to enhance the flow of *qi* (an ancient term given to what is believed to be vital energy) in the body, improve blood circulation, and enhance immune function.

Reiki: Reiki is a Japanese word meaning universal life force energy. Reiki is based on the belief that when spiritual energy is channeled through a Reiki practitioner, the patient's spirit is healed, which in turn heals the physical body.

Therapeutic touch: Therapeutic touch is derived from an ancient technique called laying-on of hands. It is based on the premise that it is the healing force of the therapist that affects the patient's recovery; healing is promoted when the body's energies are in balance, and by passing their hands over the patient, healers can identify energy imbalances.

Naturopathic physicians are doctors trained in conventional medicine as well as herbology, supplements, and diet. **Herbalists** belong to an unregulated profession, so you may find a wide range of expertise available. They may use herbs singly or in combination to promote health and well-being. **Chiropractors** manipulate bones, joints, and muscles to relieve pain and restore energy. **Acupuncturists** insert needles into selected points of the body, also to relieve pain and restore balance of energy flow. **Doctors of Chinese medicine** find unique combinations of Chinese herbs and North American herbs to treat and balance complex systems of the body. **Massage therapists** use a variety of strokes ranging from light touch to deep muscle massage to relieve stress and aid in relaxation.

Herbals

Using herbs to heal has been a popular practice for thousands of years, long before the arrival of conventional medicine. Not intended as a substitute for medical opinion, herbs used appropriately can be an excellent complement to a wellness regime. Depending on the desired effect, the entire plant or parts of it is used: roots, leaves, flowers, bark, and berries. Herbs can be used individually or in combinations and can be made into teas (sometimes called by herbalists as infusions or light decoctions), salves, tinctures, or taken in pill form. *Infusion* is the process of making the tea by pouring one pint of water over one ounce of an herb and letting it stand, covered, for twenty minutes. *Light decoction* is the process of extracting the essential ingredients from the thicker leaves and seeds of the herb by simmering the plants in water for five minutes, then steeping them in a covered pan for fifteen to thirty minutes. A *tincture* is a concentrated extract made by soaking ground herbs in a solvent (alcohol) and water and then pressing out the liquid. Sometimes glycerin is added after removing the alcohol to make an alcohol-free liquid extract.

Herbs work in a gentler and more gradual fashion than pharmaceuticals, which give quick but temporary relief. Generally herbs need to be taken in large quantities for a long period of time before the beneficial effects are felt. Your herbalist or naturopath will be able to recommend the appropriate amount of time and dosage. Most herbs are very safe, but there are some cautions. According to Brenda Beeley, author of *A–Z Guide to Natural Healing*, "some herbs are potentially harmful when used improperly or in excessive amounts . . . such as chaparral, comfrey root, and ma huang (ephedra)."

Hobbs concurs by saying that modern science has identified alkaloids in comfrey and chaparral that stress the liver. Children, pregnant women, and people with preexisting liver conditions should avoid this herb altogether. Ephedra contains a potent plant alkaloid called ephedrine. Alkaloids are natural plant chemicals that contain nitrogen as part of their structure. "Because of its ability to give many users an extra jolt of energy and possibly melt away unwanted fat, the herb has seen sales increases . . . over the last ten years. . . . Side effects include disturbed sleep, nervousness, anxiety, heart palpitations, etc.," Hobbs says. The American Heart Association urged a ban on all ephedra products in 2003.

Common wisdom is that no one herb helps everyone. Try several until you find the one for you. If you experience discomfort with any herb, discontinue it immediately.

Herbs for Sleep

Note: Because all bodies are different the dosage of these herbs depends on the severity of symptoms, weight, age, and response of the individual.

California Poppy

The bright orange root is the strongest medicinal part of this plant, but the leaves and flowers are also used. Some say it works best the second or third night taken in tea or tineture form.

Catnip

A member of the soothing mint family, catnip grows like a weed in the United States and Europe. While it excites cats, it produces the opposite results in humans. It is used as a mild tea for calming, sweat-releasing, and digestion-promoting effects.

Chamomile

Perhaps the most commonly known sleep aid, chamomile flowers are made into tea all over the world. The herb is called *manzanilla* in Spain and Latin America. Drink it liberally as a tea; it can also be made into a cream for skin irritations, burns, and bites.

Hops
The female cones of this plant produce a yellow powder, which can be processed for medicinal reasons and for brewing beer. Take it in capsule, tincture, or tea form.

Kava Kava
A product of the pepper family, kava kava (also known simply as "kava") is a rapidly acting herb, which can be taken in capsule, tincture, or tea form. It is also useful for stress and anxiety reduction. The NCCAM has recently released a consumer advisory on kava, citing safety as a concern. People, especially those with liver disease or liver problems, or who are taking drugs that can affect the liver, should talk with their health-care practitioner before using kava.

Lavender
Easy to grow in your garden, this Mediterranean plant sprouts fragrant, colorful, and delicate flowers atop leggy stems. When the flowers open in early summer, cut the stalks, tie them in small bunches and hang them upside down in a dry place out of direct sunlight. A delightful sleep enhancer, the dried flowers can be strewn into your hot bubble bath, or placed in small muslin bags and into your pillowcase. Lavender in the form of essential oil can be used in your bath as well.

Lemon Balm
A fast-growing and hardy plant from the soothing mint family, lemon balm can be made into teas or tinctures. The dried leaves can also be used in aromatherapy preparations.

Passion Flower
This native North American vine was used by the Aztecs as a sedative and pain killer. The whole plant is used in tinctures, capsule,

or tea form. It may be especially effective when combined with other herbs like California poppy and valerian.

Saint-John's-wort
Gaining popularity as an alternative to pharmaceutical anti-depressants, Saint-John's-wort is available in tincture and capsule form. In cream form, it is also effective for skin irritation.

Skullcap
A member of the mint family, skullcap is native to eastern North America and was used by Indians for its calming effects. It has also been effectively used as an aid to alcohol, tobacco, and drug withdrawal.

Valerian Root
Valerian was widely recommended by ancient Greek physicians and is currently used in many cultures as a mild sedative and tranquilizer. It is a perennial that grows wild in woodlands, along river banks, and in damp meadows all over Europe. The root of the plant is used medicinally for insomnia and anxiety, as well as a general sedative. Extracts of valerian root are commonly combined with other mildly sedating herbs like passion flower, lemon balm, and hawthorn. Concerning interactions with other herbs and supplements, the *Natural Medicines Comprehensive Database* reports that the use of valerian with other herbs and supplements that have sedative properties might enhance its therapeutic value but could possibly have adverse effects. Some of these products include calendula, California poppy, catnip, celery, Siberian ginseng, German chamomile, goldenseal, gotu kola, hops, kava, L-tryptophan, melatonin, sage, Saint-John's-wort, sassafras, shepherd's purse, skullcap, stinging nettle, and wild carrot. Its nonaddictive properties make it a logical alternative to the potentially addictive benzo-diazepene class of drugs such as Halcion. Dr. Northrup reports

that is has a very bad taste, so she recommends taking it in capsule form.

Combination Herbs

A recommended herbal formula for inducing sleep is:

> Mix 1 teaspoon of each of the following in 4 cups of water: Valerian root, kava root, linden flowers, chamomile flowers, and catnip leaf. Bring herbs and water to a boil, then simmer the mixture for 20 minutes. Drink 1 cup of the tea, 2 to 3 times daily before meals. Or, mix 1 teaspoon each of the individual tinctures in 1 cup of water and drink ½ cup, 2 times daily.

> Example of a tincture using lavender:
> Add approximately 7 ounces of dried lavender flowers to ⅔ of a quart of glycerol (a syrupy alcohol also called glycerin, available in health-food stores) and ⅓ quart of water. Or use 1 cup brandy or vodka and 3 cups of water. Cover for two weeks. To induce sleep, take 1 teaspoon after dinner and 2 to 3 teaspoons at bedtime.

Other Herbs

Melatonin

Humans naturally produce melatonin, which is a hormone secreted by the brain's pineal gland. Not to be confused with melanin, (skin pigment) melatonin produces drowsiness and is affected by lightness and darkness, shift work, jet lag and depression. In that regard melatonin is useful if you have to reset your biological clock due to shift work or travel across time zones. The amount of melatonin we produce changes with age, particularly after age 70. Dr. Hauri reports that in larger doses (3–5 mg) melatonin actually may have a sedative effect and induce sleep in some patients, especially those who have a melatonin deficiency, as occurs frequently in the elderly. It is either synthetically produced or extracted from bovine pineal glands. As with any sleeping pill, Dr. Hauri recommends that if you use melatonin, consult your physician and use it infrequently and in as low a dosage as possible.

L-tryptophan

Past studies have demonstrated the beneficial effects of L-tryp-tophan, an amino acid found in such common foods as meat, dairy products, beans and leafy green vegetables. Before 1989, supplemental doses of L-tryptophan were advised for those suffering from insomnia. The thought was that the amount of L-tryptophan found in common foods was too small to have a significant affect on your sleep. However, the FDA removed L-tryptophan from the market after it was found to contain toxic contaminants from the manufacturing process. Subsequent studies indicate that large amounts of L-tryptophan taken separately can still pose serious health hazards. Since no one is known to have suffered from an old-fashioned glass of warm milk, it may be best to trust mom's advice and return to this natural source of the drug. L-tryptophan rich foods eaten before bed can help promote restful sleep, such as turkey, milk, tuna, eggs, fish, almonds, bananas, or peanut butter. And ice cream!

5-HTP

Natural 5-HTP comes from the seed of a legume grown in Africa, and synthetic versions are on the market, which appear to have the same biological effects. It is basically an amino acid that is a metabolite, or naturally occurring compound of L-tryptophan.

Foods containing L-tryptophan have sleep inducing qualities. 5-HTP is most frequently used for insomnia, appetite control, and mood enhancement, but also may play a role in managing depression, anxiety, and PMS, among other disorders. Consult an herbalist for the correct dosage.

Aromatherapy

Your sense of smell can serve you well by alerting you when things are spoiled and thus inedible and by reminding you of pleasant memories such as your mom's freshly baked chocolate chip cookies. The science of smell, or *aromatherapy*, is based on calling forth pleasant memories. Whole industries heavily rely on luring customers through the use of smell, such as candle shops and grocery stores. Hobbs in *Herbal Remedies for Dummies* devotes an entire chapter to aromatherapy, saying that:

> Scratching a eucalyptus fruit and inhaling deeply for a
>   moment sharpens memory and alertness, and gives
>   a feeling of safety;
> A sprig of rosemary helps settle emotions down;
> Lavender enhances creativity and lifts the spirits.

The aromas you choose may come to you in the form of plants, flowers, or essential oils, which are superconcentrated and the most effective. You can put a few drops of the oil into very hot water and tent a towel over your head to help you inhale the steam. Small amounts of the oils are usually safe applied directly to your skin, although some people may experience redness and irritation because of the high concentration of the oil. You can dilute an essential oil, such as lavender (¼ teaspoon) with a fixed oil like sweet almond oil (6 tablespoons). You can also buy inhalers of popular scents or diffusers, which dispense the essential oil into the air by means of vibration or heating.

The most popular essential oils for insomnia are chamomile, lavender, and vetiver. We've discussed chamomile and lavender above. Vetiver is an earthy and spicy-scented oil that is also beneficial to arthritis and tight muscles.

Homeopathy

The key to homeopathy's process is to find the remedy that most closely matches the symptoms the person presents. This basic "like cures like" method of healing is based on the principle that a small amount can relieve symptoms that a larger amount of the same substance creates. Brenda Beeley's example is this: "While a physician would have you take an antihistamine to dry up your runny nose and watery eyes (and make you sleepy and dry-mouthed), a homeopath might recommend you try *Allium cepa*, or onion, which anyone who cooks will recognize as inducing copious eye tearing and a drippy nose." But the minute amount of it actually works like the antihistamine without the side effects. Homeopathy is safe and easy to give in tiny sweet-tasting pill form to children and infants, as well as adults. The following is a list of possible remedies for the different reasons that cause insomnia:

Nux vomica
Gelsemium
Chamomilla
Avena sativa
Coffea cruda
Ignatia
Pulsatilla
Aconite
Lycopodium
Socculus
Arnica

Opium
Arsenicum
Rhus
Aurum

For a remedy to work most effectively, it is important not to eat or drink anything twenty minutes before and after a remedy is given.

Consult a homeopathic practitioner for the remedy most appropriate for your symptoms. Your local health foods store will likely have a list of practitioners in your area.

Chinese Medicine

Chinese medicine evolved five thousand years ago from the philosophy of Daoism. People who practice Daoism are great listeners of nature and feel that you can't listen very well if things are "covered up" by drugs. The basic goal of Chinese medicine is to bring a person into balance. Altogether it means "Moving toward balance by grabbing the Chi." The two polar principles of Chinese medicine are yin and yang, and disease is an imbalance in these principles. It is possible to describe every aspect of the body in terms of yin and yang, and to do so, the body is divided into five key systems:

Organ	Tissue	Sense	Spirit	Emotion
Kidneys	bones/head hair	hearing	will	fear
Liver	sinews	sight	ethereal soul	anger
Spleen	flesh	taste	thought	thinking/worry
Lungs	skin/body hair	smell	corporeal soul	grief/sadness
Heart	blood vessels	speech	spirit	joy/fright

Source: *Curing Insomnia Naturally with Chinese Medicine* by Bob Flaws

To help make a diagnosis, practitioners of Chinese medicine look at patterns one displays on a person's tongue and taking a pulse. An example of a pattern for insomnia would be heart/blood stasis: the kidney naturally goes into a yin deficiency state around the age of forty-nine. Menopause is heart/yin deficiency, directly connected to the kidney, so if there is steady insomnia and/or menopause, the treatment would be to nourish the kidney, calm the mind, and clean the empty heart with acupuncture or herbal medicine made up of ginseng plus thirteen Chinese herbs. This is called a protocol formula, which might be further customized to meet the needs of the person, in contrast to the tendency of Western medicine to simply put women on estrogen.

Practitioners incorporate herbals, diet, exercise, massage, and acupuncture into their treatment regime.

Acupuncture

Acupuncture has attracted widespread attention in this country as a method to treat insomnia only in the past few years. This is ironic in that acupuncture is one of the most ancient of medical treatments, possibly dating from 2000 B.C. The American Academy of Medical Acupuncture reports that over the past two thousand years, more people have successfully been treated with acupuncture for a variety of ailments than with all other health modalities combined.

The term acupuncture is derived from the Latin *acus* (needle) and *punctura* (puncture), and was coined by Jesuit missionaries returning to Europe from China in the sixteenth century. As its name implies, this medical art involves the insertion of needles through the skin into very precise points in the body. The needles employed are very thin and solid, and are made from stainless steel. The point is smooth and insertion through the skin is not as painful as injections or blood sampling. Most patients feel only minimal pain as the needles are inserted; some feel no pain at all. Generally, once the needles are in place, patients feel no pain.

The Chinese theory behind acupuncture explains that the body's vital energy, known as *chi* or *qi,* moves along designated channels sometimes called "meridians," each of which is governed by a major body organ. These channels may be thought of as rivers that flow through the body to nourish the tissues. When a river is obstructed, the energy is backed up in one part of the body and restricted in others. Acupuncture points are located along the meridians and needling of these points alters the flow of energy in the system. Acupuncture thus influences the meridians by unblocking obstructions and restoring balance, allowing energy to flow freely again.

Acupuncture is a time-honored treatment for insomnia in China and in other parts of east Asia. Traditionally, Chinese medicine views all sleep disorders as stemming from either a deficiency in *qi* or a surplus of *qi* in body organs—mainly, the kidney and heart. Treatments based on this model have yielded impressive results. In a 1995 article published in the medical journal *Psychiatry and Clinical Neurosciences,* Chinese researchers reported a 90 percent "effectiveness rate" of acupuncture treatment for insomnia.

Western scientists have sought a more quantifiable and biochemical explanation for acupuncture's effectiveness. So far, no single model has proven adequate, but acupuncture does cause at least two significant effects, which may play a role. First, needling acupuncture points causes an increased release of endorphins and enkephalins (the body's natural opiate-like painkillers) into the bloodstream. Some studies have suggested that insomnia may be due in part to a deficiency of endorphins, lending to the plausibility of this explanation. Second, it has also been shown that acupuncture alters the regulation of certain neurotransmitter chemicals within the body and brain. These chemicals allow communication between neurons—the cells that govern the function of your brain and nervous system. Among a multitude of other functions, neurotransmitters help to regulate the sleep-wake cycle. For instance, neurotransmitters in the brain facilitate and regulate the release of melatonin (which helps us sleep) from the hypothalamus and cortisol (which helps us wake up) from the adrenal gland.

An examination of the use of acupuncture for insomnia reveals some interesting similarities as well as some contrasts to the use of medication. For example, like medication, acupuncture causes significant quantifiable biochemical changes within the body. However, acupuncture does not typically cause lingering side effects and does not lead to the buildup of toxic metabolites (breakdown products) within the body or the brain. Unfortunately, side effects and the buildup of metabolites are often the consequence of sleep medication, depending, of course, on the specific drug in question.

Many medications used to initiate or prolong sleep also result in daytime sluggishness and fatigue. The longer the half-life of the drug, the greater the risk. For more details, please refer to chapter 13 on the use of medication for sleep disorders.

Acupuncture is likely to be much less dramatically effective in inducing sleep in the short term, but its effects tend to be cumulative over time. This profile is in stark contrast to that of medication, which can exert dramatic, immediate effects but may become less effective over time because of the development of tolerance and/ or dose-limiting side effects.

Finally, where insomnia is concerned, acupuncture is similar to medication in one particularly important way: both are most effective when used in concert with other strategies. Such strategies are outlined in detail in this book and include useful ways of altering one's environment, diet, behavior, and thought processes.

Unfortunately, acupuncture does not always work for everyone. Factors associated with the success or failure of acupuncture include medications, which may influence or interfere with its effects; the specific chemical makeup of an individual patient and his physiologic response to needling; as well as the skill and experience of the acupuncture practitioner. No specific acupuncture treatment has been found to be consistently superior to any other in terms of combating insomnia. A treatment protocol will depend on the practitioner's prior training and experience, as well as an evaluation of the patient's specific sleep and related health problems. Acupuncture treatments, by necessity, are individualized to each patient.

If you do decide to pursue a course of acupuncture as part of your approach to overcome insomnia, ensure that you are working with a licensed practitioner. Appropriate practitioners may include both physicians and nonphysicians. Licensure regulations vary from state to state, but nonphysician acupuncturists must pass a standardized exam and be accredited by a national licensing board. Properly trained and certified nonphysician acupuncturists bear the title L.Ac. (licensed acupuncturist). Physicians generally must be licensed to practice acupuncture by their state medical boards. An up-to-date listing of physicians with specialized acupuncture training can be found on the American Academy of Medical Acupuncture's Web site, www.medicalacupuncture.org, which is also a good resource for information on acupuncture in general.

Before starting treatment, inquire about a practitioner's experience in treating sleep disorders. Acupuncturists, like all health-care professionals, have different clinical interests and areas of expertise. When you arrive at the office or clinic, don't be surprised if the practitioner asks to examine your tongue or feel the pulses in your wrists—these are important parts of a traditional Chinese medical examination that many acupuncturists incorporate in their evaluation. Above all, make sure that your acupuncturist is a good listener who takes the time to understand your unique sleep and health history.

Acupressure

Just as acupuncture works to balance the flow of *qi,* acupressure uses the same or similar meridian system to release blocked *qi.* As its name implies, pressure is applied to these points by rubbing or kneading with the fingers and hands. Shiatsu is a particular type of acupressure developed by the Japanese from the original Chinese techniques. The *Alternative Medicine Definitive Guide to Sleep Disorders* describes shiatsu this way:

> Shiatsu uses a sequence of firm rhythmic pressure applied to specific points for 3–10 seconds and, like acupuncture, is designed to awaken, calm, and harmonize the meridians. Shiatsu affects not only the acupressure point, but the entire mind and body, making it one of the most effective forms of bodywork for sleep disorders.

Massage

The health benefits of massage are prolific and legendary. Rapidly gaining in popularity and respect as an important addition to conventional medical techniques, massage does the following as an aid to sleep:

- helps relieve pain and reduce swelling
- improves both blood flow and lymphatic circulation
- promotes relaxation
- reduces muscle soreness and spasm
- helps correct posture
- helps eliminate toxins from the body

The *Alternative Medicine Definitive Guide to Sleep Disorders* reports, "Lymphatic massage, for example, can move metabolic waste through the body to promote a rapid recovery from illness or disease. Other studies show that massage can be used as an adjunct in the treatment of cardiovascular disorders and neurological and gynecological problems, and can often be used in place of pharmacological drugs."

The following massage technique can be used at home with a partner and is enthusiastically recommended by Shalom Vegodsky, health consultant and energy kinesiologist. Brought to us by Arlene Green, who teaches self-help techniques for reducing stress and pain, both Green and Vegodsky claim this technique to work within minutes.

Brazilian Toe Massage

Green comments that this technique was originally presented in 1980 at a Touch for Health International Convention by a Brazilian named José De Aragao. It involves holding the toes very lightly in the sequence described below. To quote Green, "Some say this technique affects acupuncture energy as one connects up various end points of meridians while holding the fingers to the toes. Others believe that it works with polarity principles as the fingers and toes alternate positive and negative electrical charges."

The technique deeply relaxes the body, so make sure that you are in a comfortable position that you can maintain for about fifteen minutes.

Procedure:

1. Lie down in a comfortable position on your back.
2. Have your partner stand or sit at your feet so that your toes can be easily held without straining.

3. The toes are held very lightly, both feet at the same time in a specific sequence (see chart).

4. Hold each set of toes for three minutes, fingers on top of toenail, thumb always on the bottom (under the pad).

5. Change after three minutes, moving the thumb then the fingers to the next toe very smoothly and gently.

Feet *Toe #*	*Your Hands* *Thumb and Finger*
3 (middle)	T + middle
4	T + ring
5 (baby)	T + pinkie
2	T + index
1 (big)	T + index and middle*

*Hold each side of base of nail.

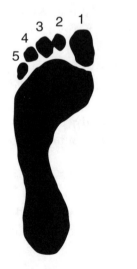
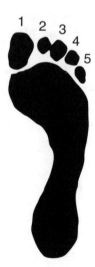

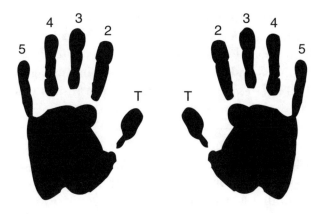

Yoga

Yoga is an ancient Eastern practice promoting mind/body unity. It combines the spiritual practice of meditation with the physical practice of deep breathing and postures, also known as poses. Hatha yoga is probably the most well known type of yoga in the West, and generally has twelve postures designed to maintain basic physical health and fitness. Posture is very prominent among all the varieties of yoga practice in general. Hatha yoga emphasizes breath, however, as the link between mind and body. As breath slows down, so do thoughts and emotions. This is helpful for promoting sleep, because as you concentrate on your breathing, you learn to hold your restless mind in check.

You also learn to disengage your senses from the outer world, and focus your mind on a single thing, be it a thought, mental image, sound (such as the mantra "om"), a bodily locus (such as the third eye or the heart) or even an external object such as a statue of a sacred figure or flame of a candle.

Today Westerners often practice yoga techniques (especially postures) apart from the spiritual origins of Hinduism, Buddhism and Jainism, native to India. While the postures are very effective for maintaining and even restoring one's physical health, practitioners claim the true power of yoga lies in its potency as a path to lasting happiness and inner freedom. Yoga has no age limit and people of all ages experience positive health results through the practice of postures, breathing and meditation.

For more information on CAM or NCCAM, contact the NCCAM Clearinghouse at 1-888-644-6226, toll free; 301-519-3153; TTY 1-866-464-3615, for deaf or hard-of-hearing callers. E-mail: info@nccam.nih.gov. Web site: nccam.nih.gov. Address: NCCAM Clearinghouse, P.O. Box 7923, Gaithersburg, MD 20898-7923.

15

Most Sedating
Things to Do
While Awake

If you faithfully follow the stimulus control procedures outlined in chapter 5, you will at first find yourself sitting up, staring at the walls, and wondering what to do. When this happens, it's a good idea to have a plan. If you organize two or three things you can do while awake, the prospect of getting out of bed won't be so distasteful. You'll have something to look forward to. Of course, you don't want to do anything *too* interesting or stimulating, since the idea is to lull yourself back to sleep.

Ideal activities are those you can begin and end as you choose, so that when you feel sleepy you can put what you're doing aside and go back to bed. A book of short stories might be perfect for you. An activity to *avoid* would be an exciting movie that you just *have* to see to the end.

Since a common trait among insomniacs is obsessiveness and compulsiveness, be aware of your tendency to want to complete your projects perfectly. Avoid becoming anxious about your night-time activities. Carefully choose projects that will help you slow down, not speed up.

Insomnia researcher Dr. Michael Colligan wrote in *Creative Insomnia* that when faced with time to kill, you may as well consider it "found" time and enjoy it. He offers lists of things to do, ranging from stargazing to figuring your biorhythms. With his suggestions and the help of others, I have put together a suggested list of the Dozen Most Sedating Things To Do While Awake. These are only suggestions; as you read through them, they may trigger your own unique ideas.

1. Read
   The wee hours are a great time for reading, provided, of course, that what you read isn't so exciting that it makes you want to stay awake until you get to the end. Read those classics you meant to get to in high school or college but never found the time. Or read nonfiction. Are you interested in history? Gardening? Antiques? Or choose self-help books or books on spiritual subjects. These can give you a feeling of well-being and a sense that there are solutions to life's problems, plus you can read short amounts at a time.
   If you have a bedmate, you might also consider purchasing a bed light, a small type of flashlight that runs on batteries and that can be attached to your book or easily held. This way you can read without disturbing the person next to you.
   The following are books written specifically for insomniacs:
   Night: Night Life, Night Language, Sleep, and Dreams. A. Alvarez. W. W. Norton and Company, New York, 1995.
   The Literary Insomniac: Stories and Essays for Sleepless Nights. Elyse Cheney and Wendy Hubbert, eds. (New York: Doubleday, 1996).
   Insomnia Poems: Acquainted with the Night. Lisa Russ Spaar, ed. (New York: Columbia University Press, 1999).
   Hello Midnite: An Insomniac's Literary Bedside Companion. Deborah Bishop and David Levy. New York: Touchstone Books, Simon and Schuster, Inc., 2001.

And for those hot-flash nights, a lighter look at
menopause:
Menopaws (The Silent Meow). Martha Sacks. (Berkeley:
Ten Speed Press, 1995).
2. Keep a journal.
Keep a notebook and pen or pencil by your bedside to
record any dreams you might recall, troubling thoughts,
or any thoughts at all. It can sometimes be soothing just
to put down on paper what you are thinking. If anxious
thoughts are crowding out your mind, just the act of recording those thoughts can put some distance between
you and them, allowing you the space to sleep. Plus, if
you are looking at dream meanings, you'll have a better
chance at recalling the dream characters and situations if
they are recorded shortly after you experience the dream.
Also check out chapter 8 for more information on dream
journals.
3. Collect, cut, and organize coupons.
If you like saving grocery money by using coupons, use
the nighttime to throw out expired ones and organize the
current ones. Put them into food groups. Devise a coupon
holder so that they stay neat and retrievable.
4. Organize your recipe box and/or sort the tool box. Separate nails from screws, ratchets from wrenches.
How many times have you gone thumbing through your
recipe box searching for that out of place recipe while
the water's boiling over and your hands are full of egg-
plant? Here's a perfect opportunity to once and for all
throw out those recipes you will *never* use and put into
order those you will. Rewrite well-loved recipes that are
now splattered and stained. Put clear protective tape over
those you plan to use regularly. Or put them behind plas-
tic or in a photo album for protection and easy location.

5. Remove your name from junk-mail lists.
   Always a wish of many people, but unfortunately low on
   the priority list. Here's your chance to make it clear to
   vendors that you do not want their paper stuffing your
   mailbox, their callous cold-call voices in your ears, or
   their internet pop-up ads. Do one or all of the following:
   a. Write to magazines you subscribe to. Ask them *not* to
      disclose your name or address to other services. This
      is the number one way your name gets out.
   b. Collect all junk mail for one or two months. Systemati-
      cally write to each and every vendor requesting that
      they remove your name from their list. Use the postage
      paid-envelope that came with the junk mail. That way
      the vendor will be paying for the message you are send-
      ing, not you.
   c. Get a copy of Form 2150 from the U.S. Post Office
      and list all the vendors on the form whose mail you
      are refusing. The post office will pull the mail before
      it is sent.
   d. The Federal Trade Commission sponsors a national
      do-not-call registry where you can register online
      or by telephone to stop telephone solicitors. To
      register for this free service, your name, address, and
      telephone number are placed on a "do-not-call" or
      "do-not-mail" file. The file is updated monthly and
      distributed four times a year, and your name remains
      on file for five years. You may register online at
      www.donotcall.gov or by calling 1-888-382-1222; TTY,
      1-866-290-4236.
6. Update your phone/address book.
   Make sure you have current numbers listed for your
   doctor(s), pharmacy, fire and police departments, and
   any other emergency services you might need.

7. Organize photos and fill albums.

   Pull out those years of photos still in their packets from the camera shop or drug store and organize them in an album.

8. Do needlework.

   Take up needlepoint, quilting, knitting, or another type of needlework that might appeal to you. Once you get the hang of it, these activities require very little active attention and can provide hours of distraction. If you still need to satisfy that compulsive part of you and don't want to take up anything new until you finish old work, then you might want to spend the wee hours sewing on buttons or mending clothes.

9. Listen to soothing music.

   There are literally hundreds of CDs available that specialize in "soothing sounds." You have a wide variety of choices ranging from ocean waves to "space" music for a new age. You can sample the sounds on the internet, if you wish. Check out amazon.com's mood music page where you can browse its relaxing music catalog containing soothing music for sleep and meditation, as well as affirmations and nature sounds. You can also visit yogamusicvideo.com, spiritvoyage.com, and serenitysupply.com.

10. Surf the net or visit chat rooms.

    Just put the words "sleep" or "insomnia" into your search engine and be amazed at the wealth of resources you'll find. For example, a pleasant late-night chat room for insomniacs can be found at awakeinphilly.com.

11. Luxuriate in a warm bath.

    Fill your bath with bubbles scented with sleep-inducing aromatic oils, such as lavender or sage. Light scented candles. Drink herbal teas especially formulated to invite sleep, such as those containing valerian root,

chamomile, or catnip. Put a few drops of lavender oil on your pillow.
12. Do your taxes. Guaranteed to induce sleep and/or infuriation.

Insomnia Tours

You might be interested to know that once or twice a year, Baltimore Rent-A-Tour conducts very popular Insomnia Tours for groups of thirty or more for night-owl fun. Beginning at 1:30 A.M., the group tours a variety of historic and cultural sights and winds up with a postsunrise breakfast. A great way to beat the traffic! Baltimore Rent-A-Tour might consider organizing an insomnia tour in your area. Call or write Baltimore Rent-A-Tour, 3414 Philips Drive, Baltimore, Maryland, 21208, 410-653-2998, or e-mail brat1974@aol.com.

Hopefully these ideas have stimulated your thinking, and you now have a plan to keep yourself occupied. Perhaps these things are so *boring* that you'd just as soon go back to sleep. In any case, know that you have options. Keep a positive attitude when you can't sleep. Consider these "extra" hours an opportunity to read that (mildly boring) book you've always wanted to read, or begin that knitting project. Staying positive and upbeat is better than being fretful. It's less stressful and much more productive.

Final Words

16

Sometimes it will seem that everything you try is fruitless, that your sleep problem relentlessly drags on with no relief in sight. You will ask yourself, "Why even bother to attempt a new technique? It will turn out to be a failure like the rest and I'll be stuck with this stupid problem for life." If you find yourself falling prey to this line of thinking, stop yourself immediately. It will do you no good whatsoever to dwell on the hopelessness of it all. This kind of self-defeating talk only promotes victimization. If you regard yourself as a victim of poor sleep, leaving yourself no avenues for change, you will remain a victim forever.

This is not to say that your sleep problem will disappear overnight if you simply adjust your attitude. Most likely it will not. But, as with any self-help maneuver, careful persistence on your part will pay off in the long run. Remember these four points when you feel despair over your sleep problem. Read them over and over to bolster your spirit and resolve.

1. Keep your expectations realistic. Allow yourself a gradual improvement in sleep. Permit yourself to develop slowly, over time, healthy sleep strategies. Reward yourself for even seemingly small gains.

2. Treat your problems holistically. Don't expect one sleep technique to "do it all." You are a complex being. Stay open to all the various aspects of your mind, body, and spirit. This means carefully examining your emotional well-being as well as your physical needs.
3. Adopt an attitude of passive concentration. Don't try so hard to fall asleep. Don't tackle every new technique with such zealous fervor that you lose sight of your intention: to turn your mind off and drift off to sleep. Learn to let go.
4. At the same time, don't give up. Be persistent. Learn to concentrate passively on your sleep strategies. This means not forcing the issue, but allowing yourself to be open to better sleep strategies. Commit yourself to healthy sleep.

If all else fails, pretend that this book is a sedative. Tell yourself that every time you read it, pick it up, even glance at it, your eyelids will begin to droop and you will yawn. My well-meaning husband, offering to read late-night drafts of this book before they were shipped off to the publisher, would begin eagerly, and what seemed like minutes later push the chapters aside, yawning, ready for bed. He is an example of a person particularly susceptible to suggestion. You, too, can develop the ability, perhaps not as dramatic, to react positively to certain cues. Keep this book by your bedside, and every time you wake up, look at it and remind yourself that you are in control, you are relaxed, and you can sleep.

Appendix A

Useful Web Sites

(*Note:* All Web sites were active at the time of publication.)

Sleep Disorder Centers

Both of the following Web sites have a map of the United States where you can click on your state to determine the sleep center closest to you.

National Sleep Foundation: www.sleepfoundation.org
The NSF is a nonprofit organization dedicated to prevention of catastrophic accidents caused by sleep deprivation and excessive sleepiness.

American Academy of Sleep Medicine: www.aasmnet.org
Contains useful links to research and professional sleep societies worldwide.

Other useful educational and noncommercial sites:

www.sleepnet.com
Also has sleep clinician links, information on sleep disorders, chat rooms, and a "sleep mall" where you can find the Snore

Store, CPAP (Continuous Positive Airway Pressure, a device for sleep apnea) world, and books, CDs, and tapes.

National Heart Lung and Blood Institute with the National Institute of Health: www.nhlbi.nih.gov
The primary NIH organization for research on sleep disorders.

Another site sponsored by the NIH as well as the National Library of Medicine is Medlineplus, www.medlineplus.gov, where you can search information on any health topic.

A site with audio capability, www.healthology.com, is a privately held New York-based online health media corporation that is a leading producer and distributor of physician-generated health and medical information on the internet.

Other Useful Sites

www.CNN.com/health

www.ivillagehealth.com

American Sleep Apnea Association:
www.asaa.org or www.sleepapnea.org

Restless Legs Syndrome Foundations:
www.rls.org

Society for Light Treatment and Biological Rhythms:
www.sltbr.org

Project of the Alternative Medicine Foundation, Inc.:
www.herbmed.org
www.naturaldatabase.com (complete description of side effects, cited studies, subscription required)

Mindbyte.net

Shuteye.net

Recommended sites for alternative medicines and dietary and herbal supplements:

NIH's National Center for Complementary and Alternative Medicine: www.nccam.nih.gov

Food and Drug Administration's Center for Food Safety and Applied Nutrition: www.cfsan.fda.gov

Appendix B

Caffeine Content of Foods, Beverages, and Over-the-Counter Drugs

Product	Serving Size	Caffeine Content (mg)
Soft Drinks		
7-UP	8 oz.	0
Barqs Diet Root Beer	8 oz.	15
Barqs Root Beer	8 oz.	15
Caffeine free Coca-Cola	8 oz.	0
Caffeine free Diet Coke	8 oz.	0
Coca-Cola	8 oz.	23
Diet 7-UP	8 oz.	0
Diet Coke	8 oz.	31
Diet Dr. Pepper	8 oz.	28
Diet Mountain Dew	8 oz.	37
Diet Pepsi	8 oz.	24

(continued)

Product	Serving Size	Caffeine Content (mg)
Soft Drinks *(continued)*		
Diet RC	8 oz.	36
Diet Sprite	8 oz.	0
Diet Sun Drop	8 oz.	46
Diet Wild Cherry Pepsi	8 oz.	24
Dr. Pepper	8 oz.	28
Mello Yello	8 oz.	34
Minute Maid Orange Soda	8 oz.	0
Mountain Dew	8 oz.	37
Mr. Pibb	8 oz.	40
Mug Root Beer	8 oz.	0
Pepsi	8 oz.	25
Pepsi ONE	8 oz.	37
RC Cola	8 oz.	36
Shasta Cola	8 oz.	45
Sprite	8 oz.	0
Sun Drop	8 oz.	42
Sunkist Orange Soda	8 oz.	28
Surge	8 oz.	35
Tab	8 oz.	47
Wild Cherry Pepsi	8 oz.	25
Functional Energy Drinks		
AMP	8.4 oz	75
Black Stallion	250 mL	80

Product	Serving Size	Caffeine Content (mg)
Functional Energy Drinks *(continued)*		
Jolt	12 oz	72
KMX	8 oz	53
Lift Plus	250 mL	36
Liptorian	250 mL	50
Red Bull	250 mL	80
Red Eye Gold	250 mL	48
Red Eye Power	250 mL	50
V	250 mL	50
Coffee		
Arizona Blue Luna Iced Coffees	8 oz.	40–50
Arizona Iced Coffees	8 oz.	40–50
Brewed, drip method	8 oz.	85
Cafe Vienna	8 oz.	90
Caffe Americano, grande	16 oz.	105
Caffe Americano, short	8 oz.	35
Caffe Americano, tall	12 oz.	70
Caffe Latte	6 oz.	90
Caffe Mocha	6 oz.	90
Cappucino	6 oz.	90
Cappucino, Amaretto	8 oz.	90
Cappucino, decaf	8 oz.	4

(continued)

Product	Serving Size	Caffeine Content (mg)
Coffee *(continued)*		
Cappucino, French Vanilla or Irish Cream	8 oz.	45–50
Cappucino, Mocha	8 oz.	60–65
Coffee	8 oz.	110
Coffee, decaf	8 oz.	5
Coffee, grande	16 oz.	550
Coffee, short	8 oz.	250
Coffee, tall	12 oz.	375
Espresso	1 oz.	90
Espresso, decaf	1 oz.	10
Instant	8 oz.	75
Orange Cappucino	8 oz.	102
Swiss Mocha	8 oz.	55
Viennese Chocolate Café	8 oz.	26

Note: The listed caffeine content is average for a standard brewed cup of coffee; certain brewing methods may increase or decrease the average caffeine content per cup.

Teas		
Arizona Iced Tea, Black Tea	8 oz.	16
Arizona Iced Tea, Green Tea	8 oz.	7.5
Arizona Iced Tea, Rx Power and Energy	8 oz.	30
Brewed, Imported Brands	8 oz.	60
Brewed, Major U.S. Brands	8 oz.	40
Iced	8 oz.	25

Product	Serving Size	Caffeine Content (mg)
Teas (*continued*)		
Instant	8 oz.	28
Lipton Brisk Iced Tea	8 oz.	6
Mistic Teas	8 oz.	17 (avg.)
Snapple Iced Tea, all kinds	8 oz.	21
Caffeinated Waters		
Aqua Blast	8 oz.	40
Aqua Java	8 oz.	25–30
Java Water	8 oz.	60
Krank 20	8 oz.	45
Nitro Water	8 oz.	28
Water Joe	8 oz.	35
Chocolate		
Baker's chocolate	1 oz.	26
Chocolate milk beverage	8 oz.	5
Chocolate-flavored syrup	1 oz.	4
Cocoa beverage	8 oz.	6
Dark chocolate, semi-sweet	1 oz.	20
Milk chocolate	1 oz.	6
Milk chocolate bar w/cappucino filling	1 oz.	20

(*continued*)

Product	Serving Size	Caffeine Content (mg)
Frozen Desserts		
Cappuccino chocolate chunk or cappuccino mocha fudge ice cream	8 oz.	8
Coffee frozen yogurt, fat-free	8 oz.	40
Coffee fudge ice cream, low fat	8 oz.	30
Coffee ice cream	8 oz.	58
Coffee ice cream, assorted flavors	8 oz.	40–60
Frappuccino bar	2.5 oz (one bar)	15
No fat coffee fudge frozen yogurt	8 oz.	85
Over-the-Counter Drugs		
Anacin	2 tablets	26
Aqua Ban	1 tablet	100
Cafergot	1 tablet	100
Caffedrine	2 capsules	200
Coryban-D	1 tablet	30
Darvon compound	1 tablet	32
Dexatrim	1 tablet	200
Dristan	1 tablet	30
Excedrin, max. strength	2 tablets	130
Fiorinal	1 tablet	40
Midol	1 tablet	32
Migralam	1 tablet	100

Product	Serving Size	Caffeine Content (mg)
Over-the-Counter Drugs *(continued)*		
Neo-Synephrine	1 tablet	15
NoDoz, max. strength; Vivarin	1 tablet	200
NoDoz, regular strength	1 tablet	100
Percodan	1 tablet	32
Permathene Water Off	1 tablet	100
Pre-Mens Forte	1 tablet	50
Prolamine	1 tablet	140
Triaminicin	1 tablet	30
Vanquish	1 tablet	33

(Reprinted with permission from the National Sleep Foundation.)

Selected References

General Information about Sleep

Dement, William C., M.D., Ph.D. *The Promise of Sleep.* New York: Delacorte Press, Random House, Inc. 1999.

Fritz, Roger, Ph.D. *Sleep Disorders: America's Hidden Nightmare.* National Sleep Alert, Inc. and Publishers Distribution Service, Grawn, Michigan. 1993.

Hauri, Peter, Ph.D. and Linde, Shirley, Ph.D., *No More Sleepless Nights,* New York: John Wiley And Sons, Inc., 1996.

Inlander, Charles B. and Moran, Cyntha K. *67 Ways to Good Sleep.* New York: Walker and Company, 1995.

Lacks, Patricia. *Behavioral Treatment for Persistent Insomnia.* New York: Pergamon Press, 1987.

Ross, Herbert, D.C., Brenner, Keri, L.Ac. and Goldberg, Burton. *Alternative Medicine Definitive Guide to Sleep Disorders.* Tiburon: AlternativeMedicine.com, Inc., 2000.

Williams, Mark, M.D., *The American Geriatrics Society Complete Guide to Aging and Health,* New York: Crown Publishers, 1995.

Stress Management

Catalano, Ellen Mohr, M.A. and Hardin, Kimeron, Ph.D. *The Chronic Pain Control Workbook*, second edition. Oakland: New Harbinger Publications, 1996.

Fanning, Patrick. *Visualization for Change*. Oakland: New Harbinger Publications, 1994.

Kabat-Zinn, Jon. *Wherever You Go There You Are: Mindfulness Meditation in Everyday Life*. New York: Hyperion. 1994.

Kabat-Zinn, Jon. *Full Catastrophe Living: Using the Wisdom of Your Body and Mind to Face Stress, Pain and Illness*. New York: A Delta Book, Dell Publishing, 1990.

McKay, Matthew, Davis, Martha and Fanning, Patrick. *Thoughts and Feelings: Taking Control of Your Moods and Your Life*. Oakland: New Harbinger Publications, 1998.

Menopause

Beeley, Brenda, L.Ac. *Menopause and Osteoporosis: A–Z Guide to Natural Healing*. San Rafael: The Menopause Center, 1998.

Goldstein, Steven R, M.D. and Ashner, Laurie. *Could it Be Perimenopause?* New York: Little, Brown and Company, 1998.

Laux, Marcus, N.D. and Conrad, Christine. *Natural Woman, Natural Menopause*. New York: Harper Collins, 1997.

Lee, John, M.D., Hanley, Jesse, M.D. and Hopkins, Virginia. *What Your Doctor May Not Tell You About Premenopause*. New York: Warner Books, 1999.

Love, Susan, M.D., *The Hormone Book*. New York: Random House, 1997.

Northrup, Christiane, M.D. *The Wisdom of Menopause*. New York: Bantam Books, 2001.

Walsleben, Joyce, and Rita Baron-Faust. *A Women's Guide to Sleep.* New York: Times Books, 2000.

Journals and Magazines

The American College of Obstetricians and Gynecologists' Guide to Managing Menopause. Washington, D.C. Spring/Summer, 2003.

The North American Menopause Society. *The Menopause Guidebook.* Cleveland: 2001.

Alternative Medicine: "Grow Your Own Healing Herbs", p. 72. Tiburon: Alternative Medicine, April 2003.

Bootzin, R. R. and Epstein, O. R. "Stimulus Control Instructions." In K. L. Lichstein and L. M. Morin (eds.), *Treatment of Late-Life Insomnia,* pp. 167–184, Thousand Oaks, CA: Sage, 2000.

Dreaming

Koch-Sheras, Phyllis, Ph.D. and Sheras, Peter, Ph.D. *The Dream Sharing Sourcebook.* Los Angeles: Lowell House, 1998, 1999.

Mazza, Joan, M.S. *Dreaming Your Real Self.* New York: A Perigee Book, The Berkley Publishing Group, 1998.

Van De Castle, Robert L., Ph.D. *Our Dreaming Mind.* New York: Ballantine Books, 1994.

Complementary and Alternative Medicine

Flaws, Bob. *Curing Insomnia Naturally with Chinese Medicine.* Boulder: Blue Poppy Press, Inc. 1997.

Herschoff, Asa, N.D., *Homeopathic Remedies.* New York: Avery, a member of Penguin Putnam, Inc., 2000.

Hobbs, Christopher, L.Ac. *Herbal Remedies for Dummies.* New York: Hungry Minds, Inc., 1998.

Hoffmann, David. *The Completely Illustrated Holistic Herbal.* New York: Barnes and Noble, Inc. 1996.

Natural Health: *Yoga at Home.* Boca Raton: American Media Mini Mags, Inc. 2003.

Weil, Andrew, M.D., *Self Healing.* Watertown: Thorne Communications, Inc. 2003.

Index

242   *Index*